Recent Advances in

Surgery
30

Edited by

I. Taylor MD ChM FRCS FMedSci FRCPS(Glas) Hon ILTM

Vice-Dean and Director of Clinical Studies
David Patey Professor of Surgery, Royal Free and University College London
Medical School, University College London, London, UK

C. D. Johnson MChir FRCS

Reader and Consultant Surgeon, University Surgical Unit, Southampton
General Hospital, Southampton, UK

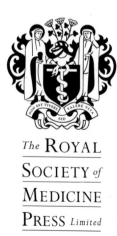

The ROYAL
SOCIETY *of*
MEDICINE
PRESS *Limited*

© 2007 Royal Society of Medicine Press Ltd

Published by the Royal Society of Medicine Press Ltd
1 Wimpole Street, London W1G 0AE, UK
Tel: +44 (0)20 7290 2921
Fax: +44 (0)20 7290 2929
Email: publishing@rsm.ac.uk
Website: www.rsmpress.co.uk

British Library Cataloguing in Publication Data
A catalogue record for this book is available from the British Library
ISBN 978–1–85315–720–2

Distribution in Europe and Rest of World:

Marston Book Services Ltd
PO Box 269, Abingdon
Oxon OX14 4YN, UK
Tel: +44 (0)1235 465500
Fax: +44 (0)1235 465555
Email: direct.order@marston.co.uk

Distribution in the USA and Canada:

Royal Society of Medicine Press Ltd
c/o BookMasters Inc
30 Amberwood Parkway
Ashland, OH 44805, USA
Tel: +1 800 247 6553/+1 800 266 5564
Fax: +1 419 281 6883
Email: order@bookmasters.com

Distribution in Australia and New Zealand:

Elsevier Australia
30-52 Smidmore Street
Marrikville NSW 2204, Australia
Tel: +61 2 9517 8999
Fax: +61 2 9517 2249
Email: service@elsevier.com.au

Editorial services and typesetting by GM & BA Haddock, Ford, Midlothian, UK

Printed in Great Britain by Bell & Bain, Glasgow, UK

Recent Advances in

Surgery
30

Recent Advances in Surgery 29
Edited by C. D. Johnson & I. Taylor

ISBN 1-85315-692-2
ISSN 0143 8395

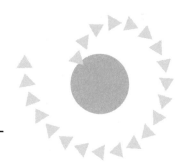

Contents

Contents

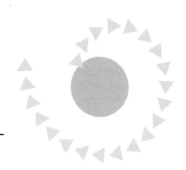

Contributors

Sayed Aly PhD FRCS
Consultant Vascular and Endovascular Surgeon, Mater University Hospital, Dublin, Ireland

Thomas Armstrong PhD MRCS(Ed)
Specialist Registrar, Department of General Surgery, Poole Hospital, Dorset, UK

Daryll M. Baker PhD FRCS
Consultant Surgeon, Department of Vascular Surgery, Royal Free Hampstead NHS Trust, London, UK

Stephen G.E. Barker MS FRCS
Senior Lecturer in Surgery, University College London, Gower Street, London, UK

Stephen J. Beningfield MB ChB FF Rad (D) SA
Division of Radiology, University of Cape Town Health Sciences Faculty, Cape Town, South Africa

José A. Cid Fernández DM FRCS
Specialist Registrar, Professorial Unit of Surgery, Nottingham City Hospital, Nottingham, UK

Philip J. Drew BSc MD MS FRCS(Eng.) FRCS(Ed.) FRCPS(Glasg.)
Professor, Hull York Medical School, Castle Hill Hospital, Cottingham, Hull, UK

Rovan E. D'Souza FRCS(Glasg.) MS DNB
Senior Clinical Fellow, Department of Vascular Surgery, Royal Free Hampstead NHS Trust, London, UK

Anthony E.B. Giddings MD FRCS
Council Member, The Royal College of Surgeons of England, London, UK

Ian Jackson MB ChB(Aberdeen) FRCA
Clinical Lead for Day Surgery, Consultant Anaesthetist, York Hospitals NHS Trust, York, UK

Colin D. Johnson MChir FRCS
Reader and Consultant Surgeon, University Surgical Unit, Southampton General Hospital, Southampton, UK

Jake E.J. Krige MB ChB FACS FRCS(Ed) FCS(SA)
Medical Research Council Liver Research Centre and Department of Surgery, University of Cape Town Health Sciences Faculty, Cape Town, South Africa

M.P. Senthil Kumar MS FRCS(Ed)
Specialist Registrar in Surgery, University College London Hospital, London, UK

Malcolm A. Loudon MD ChB FRCSEd(Gen)
Consultant Colorectal and General Surgeon, Aberdeen Royal Infirmary, Aberdeen, UK

Richard E. Lovegrove MRCS
Clinical Research Fellow, Department of Biosurgery & Surgical Technology, Imperial College London and St Mary's Hospital, London, UK

Douglas McWhinnie MD FRCS
Clinical Lead for Day Surgery, Consultant General Surgeon, Milton Keynes General Hospital NHS Trust, Eaglestone, UK

Ami Mishra MRCS
Clinical Research Fellow, Nuffield Department of Surgery, University of Oxford, John Radcliffe Hospital, Oxford, UK

James A. Pain MS FRCS
Consultant Surgeon, Department of General Surgery, Poole Hospital, Dorset, UK

Clom J. Power MD FRCS
SpR in Surgery, Mater University Hospital, Dublin, Ireland

John F.R. Robertson MD FRCS
Professor of Surgery, University of Nottingham, Nottingham City Hospital, Nottingham, UK

Sandip Sarkar MA MRCS(Glasg)
Vascular Research Fellow. Academic Division of Surgical & Interventional Sciences, University College London, London, UK

Alexander M. Seifalian PhD FInstNano
Professor, Academic Division of Surgical & Interventional Sciences, University College London, London, UK

John M. Shaw MB BCh FCS(SA)
Departmen of Surgery, University of Cape Town Health Sciences Faculty, Cape Town, South Africa

D. Mark Sibbering FRCS
Consultant Breast Surgeon, Department of Breast Surgery, Derby City General Hospital, Derby, UK

Narasimhaiah Srinivasaiah MRCS(Eng.) MRCS(Ed.) MRCPS(Glasg.) MRCSI (DNB – India)
Research Fellow, Academic Surgical Unit, Hull York Medical School, Castle Hill Hospital, Cottingham, Hull, UK

Irving Taylor MD ChM FMedSci FRCPS(Glas)
David Patey Professor of Surgery and Vice-Dean & Director of Clinical Studies, Royal Free and University College Medical School, London, UK

Paris P. Tekkis MD FRCS
Senior Clinical Lecturer and Consltant Colorectal Surgeon, Department of Biosurgery & Surgical Technology, Imperial College London & St Mary's Hospital, London, UK; and Honorary Consultant Colorectal Surgeon, Department of Colorectal Surgery, St Mark's Hospital, Harrow, UK

Eva M. Weiler-Mithoff FRCS(Ed.) FRCS(Glasg) Plast
Consultant Plastic and Reconstructive Surgeon, Canniesburn Unit, Glasgow Royal Infirmary, Glasgow, UK

A. Peter R. Wilson MA MD FRCP FRCPath
Consultant Microbiologist, Windeyer Institute of Medical Sciences, University College London Hospitals, London, UK

Ami Mishra Anthony E.B. Giddings

Risk management in surgery

1

The safety of patients was identified as an imperative for the UK in 2000 by the Department of Health's publication, *An organisation with a memory*.[1] It reported 850,000 adverse events occurring annually in NHS hospitals resulting in additional hospital days costing £2 billion a year. Adverse events are unintended, resulting from medical management rather than disease. Half of these events are thought to be avoidable and 30–50% of complications in patients undergoing surgical treatment are preventable.[2] The report followed the Institute of Medicine's *To err is human: building a safer health system*,[3] which identified four key areas for improvement: (i) a unified mechanism for reporting and analysis when things go wrong; (ii) creation of an open culture for reporting and discussion of incidents and service failures; (iii) incorporation of systems and monitoring process to enable changes; and (iv) development of a wider appreciation of the value of a systems' approach to preventing, analysing and learning from patient safety incidents. More than 5 years have passed since these problems were identified but progress has been slow.[4] The National Patient Safety Agency has established a reporting system and acted, for example to reduce confusion in drug labelling, but culture in the clinical front line has changed little. Unsafe practice, such as habitual neglect or disabling of alarms is common and associated with dangerous complacency.

Surgery is inherently unsafe and the duty of the surgeon should be 2-fold – first to minimise harm and second to maximise the benefit from care. The first has received minimal attention. The second is maintained by careful planning,

Ami Mishra MRCS
Clinical Research Fellow, Nuffield Department of Surgery, University of Oxford, John Radcliffe Hospital, Oxford, UK

Anthony E.B. Giddings MD FRCS (for correspondence)
Council Member, The Royal College of Surgeons of England, 35–43 Lincoln's Inn Fields, London WC2A 3PE, UK
E-mail: tonygiddings@btinternet.com

testing and regulation of the surgeon's training and competence. Catastrophic events in individual practice are extremely rare. By contrast, minor failures in everyday care are common and catastrophic consequences may arise from small cumulative events that individually may not be noticed.[5] Systems to identify and manage these risks may improve the safety of surgery when combined with greater awareness of their significance.

Key point 1

- Adverse events are wide-spread and cause significant human and financial costs – half of these adverse events are preventable.

IDENTIFICATION OF RISK

The traditional approach is to blame individuals after an active failure. Evidence from high-risk industries such as aviation has indicated that focusing on systems to prevent and mitigate errors is much more effective.[5] Such a 'systems' approach' recognises that errors are to be expected and must be managed. Psychology and human factors studies have identified two forms of system failures: (i) active failures which are immediate errors at the point of interaction between human and system; and (ii) latent conditions, arising from areas such as the organisation and its culture, staff training and competence, control and monitoring of practice.[6]

Most incidents occur due to an accumulation of latent conditions. Defence mechanisms should be designed to prevent latent conditions being the cause of failures, as there is usually little opportunity to influence active failures. Latent conditions may be considered multilayered: some dependent on hardware – alarms, physical barriers; some dependent on people – surgeons, anaesthetists, nurses; and some on procedures and management. However,

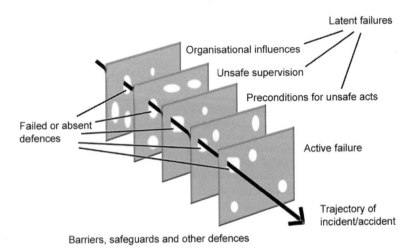

Fig. 1 James Reason's Swiss cheese model. 'Holes' in the defence mechanisms can line up, resulting in an adverse event. The alignment of the layers and their holes is constantly changing (modified from Reason[7]).

these layers have holes, and when these holes line up, the result will be an adverse event (Fig. 1).

Latent conditions (holes) can remain inactive for long periods.[7] Latent conditions include error-prone conditions in the workplace such as time pressure, understaffing, and inadequate equipment, and common, but apparently innocuous, failures in everyday practice which 'don't seem to matter'. Latent conditions are, however, more easily dealt with than active errors where it usually too late.

Key point 2

- The NHS needs to adopt a systems approach.

IDENTIFYING LATENT ERRORS IN SURGERY

It is axiomatic that efforts to prevent harm are more effective when directed to removing latent errors and as far 'upstream' as possible. Avoiding inappropriate or ineffective treatment is, therefore, a primary task.

PRE-OPERATIVE

In elective surgical cases, error can originate from the initial diagnosis or referral path. Site and side errors are eventually obvious but more visible errors, for example the urgency with which the patient needs to be seen, may not be appreciated. Delays due to referral to an inappropriate surgeon or ill-equipped hospital are not easily tracked. With more patients being referred to hospital each year, effective referral practice is even more important. The period between diagnosis and admission for treatment is made more vulnerable by interactions between several, often junior, doctors; with reduced working hours enforced by the European Working Time Directive, continuity of care is disrupted. Errors in handover are particularly common.

INTRA-OPERATIVE

The operating theatre is the most common site for adverse events in the hospital.[8] The theatre represents a point where at least three separate groups – surgeons, nurses and anaesthetists– must co-ordinate their individual efforts. Despite Kennedy's recommendations,[9] inter-professional team training has not been developed to improve this area of high risk. Operating outside one's expertise clearly contributes to risk and has been specifically identified in the General Medical Council's recent guidance.[10] Misidentification of anatomy and inexperience can increase risk but experience does not provide immunity.

Key point 3

- A just culture must be developed to ensure error reporting and provide a route to improvement.

Using video analysis, Michaelson and Levi[11] and Santora and colleagues[12] demonstrated that teamwork and communication were deficient in trauma care. In analysis of surgical procedures, Helmreich[13] has identified the same flaws, and Reader *et al.*[14] have reported teamwork skills' deficiencies in the care of intensive care patients. In a study of 48 surgical procedures in Toronto, Lingard and co-workers[15] identified failures in 30% of procedure-related communication exchanges. In an analysis of 10 complex general surgery cases, Christian *et al.*[16] identified communication breakdown as the greatest threat to patient safety in surgery. An analysis of 252 bile duct injuries following laparoscopic cholecystectomy showed that 97% were attributed not to technical errors but to misperception and an absence of corrective feedback.[17] In another study, 43% of errors in surgery reported by surgeons themselves were also due to communication failures.[18]

Recent studies at Great Ormond Street[19] and at the John Radcliffe Hospitals[20] have used a human-factors' approach to assess surgical performance. These studies confirm that the success of surgery is dependent on the effective management of resources, including team members. The findings are to be expected. Research into a series of aircraft crashes in the 1970s showed that both technical skills and non-technical skills were important. Non-technical skills are defined as the cognitive skills (situation-awareness, decision-making) and social skills (leadership, teamwork and co-operation) possessed by individuals and demonstrated by a team. They are identified by events during performance. Although separated for convenience in analysis, it must be remembered that they are, in practice, indivisible. Non-technical skills are essential to effective technical performance. Tools for assessing non-technical skills in the operating theatre have been modified from aviation. The Great Ormond Street study has shown that clinical outcome in paediatric cardiac surgery is related to the non-technical performance of the team. Studies from Oxford strongly suggest that situation awareness influences technical outcome in laparoscopic cholecystectomy.

POSTOPERATIVE

The postoperative period is often marred by complications and may reveal the effects of active adverse events. Despite knowledge of better practice and the power of focused intervention, implementation of known, better practice remains challenging.[21] For example, respiratory, urinary and wound infections are prevalent and include hospital-resistant infections. Even with policies for thomboprophylaxis, patients are disabled or killed by deep vein thromboses and pulmonary emboli.

Key point 4

- Training to develop inter-professional teamwork skills has the potential to reduce errors and improve mitigation.

THE ANALYSIS OF ERROR

An error is 'the failure of a planned action to be completed as intended (*i.e.* error of execution) or the use of a wrong plan to achieve an aim (*i.e.* error of planning)'.[9,22] Much has been learned from aviation, and as Sir Liam Donaldson has pointed out,[9] medicine should adopt these lessons. Healthcare and aviation share similar working requirements such as teamwork and both may involve high levels of physical and psychological stress.[23] Professionals in both environments experience threats from a variety of sources, which influence their risk to commit errors.[23] Aircraft accidents, though infrequent, are highly publicised and often involve huge loss of life and money. As a result, resources have been allocated over many years for the identification of causal factors. Independent investigation, public reports and rectifications are the legal and cultural norm. Research by NASA showed 70% of accidents in aviation involve human error.[13] In contrast to the drama of aircraft accidents, medical adverse events occur in individuals and are not highly visible. With no standardised method of investigation, documentation and distribution, the precise size of the problem is uncertain; however, in the UK, up to 34,000 deaths each year may be due to avoidable error.[4]

Key point 5

- No system or practice can guarantee freedom from error or its consequences.

WHAT ARE THE LESSONS FROM AVIATION?

Errors are increased by fatigue, mental overload, excessive workload, poor communication, unstructured decision-making and poor assessment and review of information available. The commission of small, non-consequential errors makes violations of technical procedures more likely.[13] Aviation has increasingly used error management strategies, including determining and teaching behaviours and attitudes that are known to prevent or mitigate error. Procedures also help, although each must be carefully implemented to avoid introducing new hazards such as compliance failures or diversion of attention from the real issues. Pilots use checklists, which reduce omission of critical steps during, for example, take-off and landing. Communication protocols, including read-back of commands, improve comprehension, help to minimise miscommunication and eliminate assumption. 'Black box' recordings enable evaluation of aviation performance, policies and processes after accidents and near misses. Finally, the aviation industry has developed a system to promote open error reporting. Employees involved in an incident must report within 24 hours and are, in general, protected from disciplinary action. The route to improvement is defined by this culture and process. It is quite different form the 'train and blame' culture of the traditional medical apprenticeship and is characterised by a much flatter professional hierarchy. Aviation has clearly shown that this is essential for safe, effective team performance. Medicine has a long way to go in improving its culture and surgery has not yet even taken on board the ergonomic lessons of workplace design which have made operating on the flight deck inherently less vulnerable to error. Operating theatres have not been significantly modified in over 40 years despite greatly increased complexity.

IMPLEMENTING RISK MANAGEMENT IN SURGERY

The essential steps are: (i) identifying latent conditions; and (ii) systems' improvement (Fig. 2).

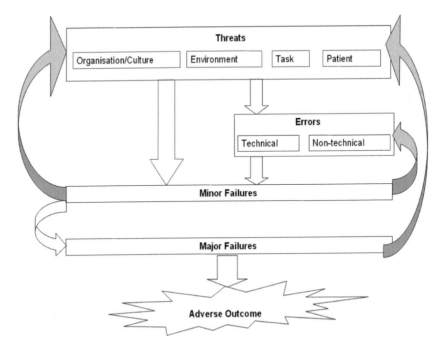

Fig. 2 Threat, error and failure model in surgery. Failures resulting from latent conditions may combine to cause active failures. Latent failures may exert their effect by contributing to an amplifying circuit.[19]

STANDARDISATION OF PROCEDURES

Standardisation is a cultural norm in delivering safety in high-reliability organisations. Standardisation simplifies key processes and reduces opportunities for error, (upstream effect). Detailed protocols are, as yet, available for only a minority of surgical procedures. Standard operating procedures (SOPs) exist for performing instrument checks and swab counts but this SOP represents the only universally accepted safety procedure in the UK.

CHECKLISTS

Currently checklists are unusual in surgery apart from the individual index cards for instruments preferred by particular surgeons. Pre-operative checklists, however, form the final assessment by anaesthetic staff prior to induction. Anaesthetic equipment has checklists, which have reduced the rate of equipment failure. Checklists could usefully be developed to assess availability and functioning of equipment in the operating theatre pre-operatively. However, they are merely a safety aid, and each individual still provides the final defence in safety issues. When checklists are used, it is important that they are compiled to fit the local context and modified where necessary by the users. All users need to be aware of the new threats introduced by the use of such lists. They may divert attention from more significant or urgent tasks or may provoke complacency. Checklists are no substitute for personal vigilance.

ERROR REPORTING AND CULTURE CHANGE

The most difficult change in safety is a requirement for a change in culture. The traditional 'train and blame' of surgical apprenticeship must be replaced by an informed culture which accepts that error, even in experts, is normal and that it must be managed openly and honestly. Punitive responses to error need to be replaced by a high-reliability response that confronts, reports and learns from error. The local culture of a unit (the way we do things around here ... when no one is looking)[24] is determined by the behaviour and practice that is deemed normal. Each member of an organisation needs to be constantly aware of their role in improving safety. A change to encouraging openness will enable reporting of mistakes and near-misses as routine. Those who report that all is not well may require support. Sir Liam Donaldson has recommended the 'creation of a culture in which quality of care and service to patients can flourish. The right culture is characterised by shared passion for quality, by openness, by support and by fairness. It is not a culture in which people are swift to blame, to find scapegoats, or seek retribution'.[25] Such motivation can be used to drive patient safety. A systems approach to risk requires a commitment at all levels of management to ensure an organisational response. Although surgeons and pilots share similarities in professional culture, doctors more readily deny the effects of stress and fatigue on decision making and performance. Pilots are more likely to disregard hierarchies in favour of teamwork.[26]

Key point 6

- Every risk-management strategy will bring its own hazards.

TEAMWORK TRAINING

Crew resource management (CRM) is a method used in aviation to focus on team performance. In aviation, CRM has promoted the breakdown of hierarchical barriers and allowed all team members to contribute to the management of a critical situation regardless of rank. Training in non-technical skills has not previously been a part of surgical training. However, attempts are being made to address this omission. First, these skills are explicitly recognised in the new Intercollegiate Surgical Curriculum Project (ISCP) and second non-technical skills courses have been developed. The Royal College of Surgeons of England has introduced such a course, *Safety and Leadership for Interventional Procedures and Surgery (SLIPS)*, and The Royal College of Surgeons of Edinburgh has commenced courses on *Non-technical skills for surgeons*. Although these are useful to teach the theory of error and its management, there is still a great deal to learn about implementation. Current

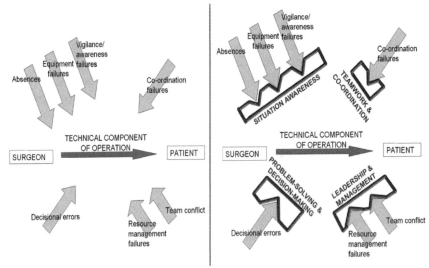

Fig. 3 Factors hindering operative performance, and how non-technical skills may improve it.

courses are aimed at surgeons and have not addressed the inter-disciplinary nature of operating theatre teamwork. No evaluation data have yet emerged on the effectiveness of these courses. At present, the courses are entirely voluntary and thus likely to attract members who embrace the concept of non-technical skills and already have a basic understanding and sympathy for the methods. The challenge is to attract cynics who lack insight to learn about matters that they consider of little relevance.

TEAMWORK AND SAFETY IN THEATRE

Research into the implementation of a programme of safety improvement is currently being conducted at the Nuffield Department of Surgery, University of Oxford. An intervention study is being performed to assess whether training in non-technical skills can improve patient outcome. The programme has been designed in conjunction with training consultants in commercial aviation. Instruction in human-factors' concepts has been combined with practical training in techniques for effective briefing, situation awareness and debriefing. This training programme has been delivered to all theatre disciplines, nurses, peri-operative practitioners and anaesthetists as well as surgeons. Technical performance is assessed with other clinical outcomes including delays, cancellations, complications and reporting of clinical incidents. Early results expose cultural and professional barriers to change in working practice and the behaviour of individuals. Agreement with the theory does not guarantee the commitment or competence to lead and embed necessary change (Fig. 3).

Key point 7

- Responsibility ultimately lies with each individual to maintain vigilance and to improve patient safety.

CONCLUSIONS

Over three decades, the ground-breaking work of human-factors' researchers working principally in the aviation industry has enabled us to aspire to parallel improvements in medicine. Human error is an inescapable fact of human behaviour; it will continue and it is, therefore, essential that secure systems to minimise the number and consequences of these errors are developed. Time, money, training and an organisational culture that encourages open-incident reporting are essential to the further development of effective systems.

Key points for clinical practice

- Adverse events are wide-spread and cause significant human and financial costs – half of these adverse events are preventable.

- The NHS needs to adopt a systems' approach.

- A just culture must be developed to ensure error reporting and provide a route to improvement.

- Training to develop inter-professional teamwork skills has the potential to reduce errors and improve mitigation.

- No system or practice can guarantee freedom from error or its consequences.

- Every risk-management strategy will bring its own hazards.

- Responsibility ultimately lies with each individual to maintain vigilance and to improve patient safety.

References

1. Department of Health. *An organisation with a memory*. London: The Stationery Office, 2000. Available at <www.dh.gov.uk/assetRoot/04/06/50/85/04065086.pdf>.
2. Healey MA, Shackford ST, Osler TM, Rogers FB, Burns E. Complications in surgical patients. *Arch Surg* 2002; **137**: 611–618.
3. Kohn LT, Corrigan JM, Donaldson MS. (eds) *To err is human: building a safer health system*. Washington, D.C.: National Academy Press, 2000.
4. Kennedy I. *Learning from Bristol: are we*? Published lecture and essay 2006. Available at <http://www.healthcarecommission.org.uk/_db/_documents/Learning_from_Bristol_a re_we.pdf>.
5. Leape LL, Bates DW, Cullen DJ. Systems analysis of adverse drug events. ADE Prevention Study Group. *JAMA* 1995; **274**: 35–43.
6. Miller LA. Safety promotion and error reduction in perinatal care. Lessons from industry. *J Perinat Neonat Nurs* 2003; **17**: 128–138.
7. Reason J. Human error: models and management. *BMJ* 2000; **320**: 768–770.
8. Leape LL. Error in medicine. *JAMA* 1994; **272**: 1851–1857.
9. Department of Health. *On the state of the public health: Annual report of the Chief Medical Officer 2005*. Available at <http://www.dh.gov.uk/assetRoot/04/13/73/67/04137367.pdf>.
10. General Medical Council *Good Medical Practice*. 2006. Available at: <http://www.gmc-uk.org/guidance/good_medical_practice/GMC_GMP_V41.pdf>.

11. Michaelson M, Levi L. Videotaping in the admitting area: a most useful tool for quality improvement of the trauma care. *Eur J Emerg Med* 1997; **4**: 59.

12. Santora TA, Trooskin SZ, Blank CA, Clarke JR, Schinco MA. Video assessment of trauma response: adherence to ATLS protocols. *Am J Emerg Med* 1996; **14**: 564–569.

13. Helmreich RL. On error management. Lessons from aviation. *BMJ* 2000; **320**: 781–785.

14. Reader T, Flin R, Lauche K, Cuthbertson BH. Non-technical skills in the intensive care unit. *Br J Anaesth* 2006; **96**: 551–559.

15. Lingard L, Reznick R, Espin S, Regehr G, DeVito I. Team communications in the operating room: talk patterns, sites of tension, and implications for novices. *Acad Med* 2002; **77**: 232–237.

16. Christian CK, Gustafson ML, Roth EM *et al*. A prospective study of patient safety in the operating room. *Surgery* 2006; **139**:: 159–173.

17. Way LW, Stewart L, Gantert W, Liu K, Lee CM. Causes and prevention of laparoscopic bile duct injuries: analysis of 252 cases from a human factors and cognitive psychology perspective. *Ann Surg* 2003; **237**: 460–469.

18. Gawande AA, Zinner MJ, Studdert DM, Brennan TA. Analysis of errors reported by surgeons at three teaching hospitals. *Surgery* 2003; **133**: 614–621.

19. Catchpole KR, Godden JR, Giddings AEB *et al*. Identifying and reducing errors in the operating theatre. *Patient Safety Research Programme Research Contract PS 012: Final Report.* 2005.

20. Mishra A, Catchpole KR, McCulloch P. Situational awareness skills may influence technical outcome in surgery. Presented at Society of Academic & Research Surgery annual meeting, 11–13 January 2006.

21. Berwick DM, Calkins DR, McCannon CJ, Hackbarth AD. The 100 000 lives campaign: setting a goal and a deadline for improving health care quality. *JAMA* 2006; **295**: 324–327.

22. Hofer TP, Kerr EA, Hayward RA. What is an error? *Effective Clin Pract* 2000; **66**: 670–676.

23. Vincent C, Taylor-Adams S, Stanhope N. Framework for analysing risk and safety in clinical medicine. *BMJ* 1998; **316**: 1154–1157.

24. Carroll JS, Quijada MA. Redirecting traditional professional values to support safety: changing organisational culture in health care. *Qual Safety Health Care.* 2004; **13**: ii16–ii21.

25. Department of Health. *Building a safer NHS for patients.* 2001. Available at <http://www.dh.gov.uk/assetRoot/04/05/80/94/04058094.pdf>.

26. Sexton JB, Thomas EJ, Helmreich RL. Error, stress and teamwork in medicine and aviation: cross sectional surveys. *BMJ* 2000; **320**: 745–749.

A. Peter R. Wilson

2

The surgical significance of MRSA

Methicillin-resistant *Staphylococcus aureus* (MRSA) was first reported in 1961 and owed its resistance to a low affinity penicillin-binding protein in the cell wall. Methicillin, the precursor of flucloxacillin, had been in general use only briefly. However, initially the organism spread slowly. There were a wide variety of strains, some of which had a brief predominance, *e.g.* 80/81. It was not until the 1990s that MRSA acquired its importance as a hospital-acquired pathogen.[1] Epidemic strains EMRSA 15 and EMRSA 16 emerged in the 1980s and spread rapidly in the late 1990s, despite infection control measures. In the UK, only 2% of strains sent to a reference laboratory were methicillin-resistant in 1990 but by 2002 43% were resistant. In some countries it became the predominant hospital pathogen forming more than 20% of all *S. aureus* isolates (US, UK, Southern Europe) while elsewhere it comprised only 5% of isolates (Northern Europe). Even within single countries, distribution was uneven. In the UK, there was a 7-fold difference in reported incidence of MRSA bacteraemia between London and the North East. The most commonly affected patients were elderly and those with surgical wounds or intravenous catheters.

Key point 1

- MRSA infection increases mortality and length of hospital stay at least 3-fold.

An increasing proportion of MRSA strains have acquired reduced susceptibility to glycopeptides, resulting in treatment failures.[2] Glycopeptide-intermediate susceptibility *Staphylococcus aureus* (GISA) can only be detected in

A. Peter R. Wilson
Consultant Microbiologist, Windeyer Institute of Medical Sciences, University College London Hospitals, 46 Cleveland Street, London W1T 4JF, UK
E-mail: peter.wilson@uclh.nhs.uk

the laboratory by additional sensitivity tests (Etest) so diagnosis is often delayed. A few isolates of vancomycin-resistant *Staphylococcus aureus* have been reported from the US. However, transmissibility and virulence appear limited.

Public and governmental pressure to reduce MRSA bacteraemia has mounted; for example, in the UK, the Department of Health has established a target of reducing incidence by 50% between 2004 and 2008. Reduction of MRSA bacteraemia requires infection control initiatives; for example, hand hygiene education and audit, screening and decolonisation before surgery, enforced protocols for safe insertion of central venous catheters and provision of alcohol hand-gel at every bedside.

PATHOGENICITY OF MRSA COMPARED WITH MSSA

Controversy remains over whether the invasiveness of MRSA exceeds that of other *S. aureus* spp. MRSA tends to colonise patients exposed to broad-spectrum antibiotics, multiple contacts and interventions. In practice, therefore, more debilitated patients are colonised and these patients subsequently develop bacteraemia. The majority of patients with MRSA infection are already colonised. Some authorities consider the likelihood of blood invasion after colonisation with MRSA is 4 times that of MSSA.[3] Additional hospital stay and mortality due to MRSA infection is significantly longer than that caused by MSSA infection.[4,5] In head and neck surgery, the cost of treatment of patients with MRSA is 3 times that of uninfected patients; in cardiac surgery, mortality is 6-fold greater.[6,7] MRSA with reduced susceptibility to glycopeptides (GISA) is increasingly encountered as a cause of bacteraemia during treatment.[2]

Both MRSA and MSSA produce factors to establish a site of infection, damage host cells, and aid spread as well as toxins producing systemic effects – coagulase, aggressins, protein A, lipase and hyaluronidase, haemolytic toxins, leukocidins, epidermolytic toxins, enterotoxins, and toxic shock syndrome toxin (TSST).

Key points 2 & 3

- MRSA is more invasive and difficult to treat than other *Staphylococcus aureus* infections.

- MRSA is spread predominantly on the unwashed hands of staff.

COLONISATION

Colonisation implies presence of MRSA at a superficial site in the absence of symptoms requiring treatment. Colonisation is usual in patients who subsequently develop infection. The nose and throat are common initial sites, either through contact with hands or inhalation of aerosol. About one-fifth of patients colonised in the perineum or elsewhere are not colonised in the nose. MRSA in wound exudate usually corresponds with infection but may represent colonisation in superficial skin ulceration.

BACTERAEMIA AND WOUND INFECTION

MRSA, like MSSA, causes a purulent infection of surgical wounds, usually associated with erythema, serous discharge and dehiscence of the wound. Abscess formation is common and deep invasion can occur, especially if a prosthesis is present. The number of bacteria required to establish a wound infection is reduced 100-fold in the presence of foreign material, whether sutures or a graft. Infection can develop following contamination of serous discharge in the early postoperative period. Once established, infection results in deep, loculated abscesses that are difficult to manage without effective drainage. When the surgical wound has passed through bone, osteomyelitis can develop requiring prolonged treatment. Osteomyelitis or endocarditis can follow bacteraemia from a wound infection but present weeks or even months after the initial infection.

TRANSMISSIBILITY

MRSA is well adapted to spreading by hand contact. The organism can survive on a surface for up to 80 days and widely contaminates the patient environment through a combination of hand contact and shed skin scales. MRSA can spread throughout a ward within a few hours of cleaning. The size of the inoculum required in establishing infection or colonisation is not known and is probably specific to the patient, depending on colonisation resistance and skin and mucosal integrity. Patients who have been treated with broad-spectrum antibiotics lack a normal body flora and are susceptible to colonisation by exogenous organisms. Prolonged hospital stay, particularly in the intensive care unit, is a major risk factor for colonisation.[8] The organism is probably seeded onto a patient's skin many times before colonisation is established. Staff, patients and their relatives disseminate MRSA throughout a ward, even if only a single carrier is present, by contact with that patient or his local environment or secondary contact with a surface or patient previously in contact with the patient.

Clothing or wristwatches of staff are also often contaminated yet allowed to come in contact with the patient's skin because they are not recognised as vectors and not frequently washed. If a patient is colonised in sputum and has a productive cough or has exfoliating skin, dissemination by airborne route can also be appreciable. Similarly, a discharging wound should not be left uncovered and dressings should be changed when strike through is observed.

HAND HYGIENE

Compliance with hand hygiene by staff is often near 20% and that by patients and relatives may be lower. Senior staff and doctors have lower hand hygiene compliance than junior staff and nurses or physiotherapists (Fig. 1).[9] Surgeons themselves pay great attention to hand hygiene in the theatre but are often responsible for poor hygiene in the ward; for example, examining wounds without removing jacket and wristwatch, washing hands or observing basic aseptic practice. Sleeves should be rolled above the elbow, wristwatch removed, the hands wetted, disinfectant applied, hands held down and all

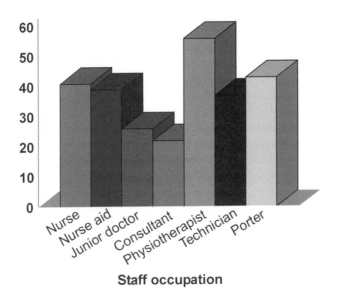

Staff occupation

Fig. 1 Hand hygiene compliance in different grades of staff.[9]

parts including the fingertips lathered. The hands are then rinsed and the tap turned off using the elbow.

Feedback on performance of hand hygiene can significantly reduce new acquisitions of MRSA in surgical wards.[10] Training on hand hygiene is, therefore, an important part of the induction of new staff.

SINGLE ROOM ISOLATION

Isolation of an MRSA-colonised patient in a single room is effective in preventing airborne dissemination and reminds staff and patients to perform hand hygiene on entering and leaving the room. Protective clothing, *e.g.* plastic aprons, is worn within the room to reduce contamination of clothing. Cleaning can be more thorough and is not compromised by transit of staff going to other beds. However, in hospitals where MRSA is endemic, the number of single rooms is usually insufficient and patients have to be isolated in the main ward. As a result, blocked hospital beds in multibed bays may be the greatest single cost in cases of infection.[11]

COHORT NURSING

Cohort nursing requires all MRSA patients in a ward to be nursed in the same bay using dedicated staff who do not nurse non-MRSA patients.[12] Accidental transmission of MRSA can then be reduced. However, cohorts do not usually apply to medical or para-medical staff and may breakdown during staff shortages or at meal times. Dedicated isolation wards, however, are effective in reducing MRSA transmission if resources exist.[13]

TRANSMISSION IN ICU

In an ICU, the high number of hand contacts and low compliance with hand hygiene is such that single room isolation does not affect the rate of acquisition of MRSA.[14] MRSA is then detectable at every bedside regardless of whether the patient is a carrier and comprises a mixture of all the strains on the unit. However, the importance of acquisition from the environment compared with that from hands is unclear.

TREATMENT

In common with wounds infected by methicillin-sensitive *S. aureus*, drainage of pus and surgical debridement are the most effective treatments. Unlike streptococcal infection, staphylococcal cellulitis tends to be localised with abscess formation. For minor superficial infections, drainage combined with topical dressings may be sufficient. Usually, however, intravenous antibiotics are necessary to prevent further spread, and bacteraemia especially during debridement. Delay in effective treatment makes subsequent cure less likely and the area of tissue loss greater.

Antibiotics commonly effective against MRSA are the glycopeptides, teicoplanin and vancomycin, and linezolid. The glycopeptides are large molecules so penetration into wounds and abscesses may be limited. These antibiotics are slowly bactericidal and may only be effective over a 24-hour period unlike the penicillins with susceptible staphylococci. Vancomycin is widely used but little has been published assessing efficacy; teicoplanin has been reported effective in 80% of cases.[15] Teicoplanin has advantages over vancomycin in that it does not require serum assay to avoid toxicity, it can be given as a once daily bolus dose and is less likely to cause red man syndrome. However, it is more expensive and requires a loading regimen of three 12-hourly doses before therapeutic levels are achieved. Linezolid has excellent penetration into all tissues whether given orally or intravenously and is active against all MRSA, including strains with reduced susceptibility to glycopeptides. However, it is very expensive and can cause thrombocytopenia and peripheral neuropathy. The manufacturers sanction use only for 28 days and then only on hospital prescription.

None of the common antibiotics used in surgical site infection are effective against MRSA including the cephalosporins and often clindamycin. Information on the use of other antibiotics such as trimethoprim is sparse. The BSAC Working Party considered tetracyclines should be more widely used on the basis of *in vitro* evidence.[15] Rifampicin or fusidic acid may be effective in combination with other agents (if active) when initial treatments have failed. Daptomycin and tigecycline are now available and potentially useful, but experience is limited.

Levels in tissue of intravenous antibiotics used in treating MRSA infection can be relatively low, especially if the abscess is large. Therefore, high doses should be used. For teicoplanin, the minimum dose should be 6 mg/kg/day and the dose of vancomycin should be determined by serum levels (trough 5–10 mg/l). Duration of treatment depends on the extent and depth of the tissue damage but should be 7–14 days. If osteomyelitis is present, treatment should be continued for 8–12 weeks combined with debridement.

Dressings are essential to keep the wound as clean as possible and to prevent further dissemination of the causative organisms. Hydrocolloids are suitable where there are low-to-moderate levels of exudate. They do not damage underlying fibroblasts and can be washed away together with the bacterial load. Alginates should be reserved for sloughy or necrotic wounds as they can be difficult to remove from cleaner wounds. Hydrocolloid or alginate dressings are usually changed every 1–2 days and accumulation of purulent material is expected. They are preferable to packing of the wound, which can result in deeper extension of the wound infection. Clear plastic dressings allow easy inspection of the wound but fluid accumulation and bacterial proliferation will occur beneath them. Fabric dressings should be reserved for relatively dry wounds and changed when strike through is observed.

Wounds with high levels of exudate may require irrigation. Drainage tubes are easier to manage than topical flushing. The mechanical action is effective in removing slough and bacteria. The use of disinfectants in the fluid is common practice but not usually necessary. Most agents are inactivated by contact with the tissues and do not penetrate the wound. Some will destroy fibroblasts necessary for wound healing. Normal saline is sufficient. Vacuum dressings have increasingly been used in recent years and are effective in promoting healing of deep cavity wounds due to MRSA. However, rigorous assessment of these dressings is relatively sparse. Sugar paste is effective in killing bacteria within a wound by its osmotic effect. It is also entirely benign towards fibroblasts and can be safely used in deep infections.

SCREENING AND TOPICAL DECONTAMINATION

Prevention of MRSA infection requires identification of the organism at carriage sites before surgery and application of topical agents to reduce the bacterial load. If started before surgery, decontamination renders surgical infection with MRSA less likely and prevents transmission of MRSA to other patients in the ward. Several studies have suggested screening and topical decontamination is effective in lowering infection, mortality rates and costs, although a Cochrane review found the evidence was not conclusive.[15,19,20] Treatment regardless of carriage status may not be effective.[21]

The usual regimen consists of mupirocin applied to the anterior nares three times a day for 5 days and chlorhexidine used daily on a sponge to apply to the skin before showering. Chlorhexidine is used as a shampoo every 2–3 days. The regimen is applied in the 5 days prior to surgery as MRSA may regrow 1–2 weeks after completion of the protocol. In the case of emergency surgery, one or more applications can be used before surgery as long as the regimen is completed after surgery. Decontamination is inexpensive but cannot be used on all patients because resistance of MRSA to mupirocin can develop.

Screening for MRSA by conventional methods takes 3 days for detection of possible carriage and another day for confirmation. Screening and decontamination can be achieved with sufficient planning in elective surgery but is unlikely to be achieved in emergency surgery. Unknown carriers can disseminate MRSA within a ward before results of screening become available. Newer, rapid methods can detect MRSA in 3–24 hours following receipt of the specimen. These methods are based on polymerase chain reaction or enzyme detection. Pre-operative screening and start of decontamination then becomes feasible in emergency surgery and reduces delays in elective surgery. However, these methods are much more expensive than conventional screening and cost reduction by prevention of infection has to be demonstrated. The average cost of a wound infection has been estimated as £4200.[22] Some hospitals only screen high-risk patients, *i.e.* those transferred from other hospitals or nursing homes or with past history of MRSA, in order to limit costs.[23] Whatever method is used, compliance with screening, transport of specimens and reporting of results have to be audited and results fedback to ensure screening is performed effectively. Patients at risk of MRSA and undergoing surgery before the MRSA result is available may have to be commenced on the decontamination protocol and discontinued if the screen later proves to be negative.

In a study of patients having surgery for proximal fracture of femur, screening and decontamination of all emergency and MRSA-positive, elective patients resulted in MRSA infection of trauma patients being reduced by 56% and of elective patients by 70%.[16] MRSA infection doubled mortality, lengthened stay by 50 days, and resulted in 19 more days of vancomycin treatment and 26 more days of vacuum-assisted closure therapy than the matched controls.

Key point 4

- Screening and topical decontamination reduces the risk of both MRSA infection in a patient and its spread to other patients.

PREVENTION OF MRSA INFECTION AT THE TIME OF SURGERY

The patient should not be admitted until the night before surgery to minimise the risk of acquisition of MRSA. Pre-assessment clinics allow routine tests and screening to be completed in advance of admission. Normal alcoholic chlorhexidine skin preparation is effective against MRSA but should be allowed to dry on the skin and not wiped off before incision. Conventional surgical prophylaxis is ineffective against MRSA. Glycopeptides are required and a single dose before the start of surgery should be adequate.[15] The dose must be sufficient to ensure adequate tissue levels (teicoplanin 6–12 mg/kg; vancomycin 1 g) and administered intravenously at the time of induction of anaesthesia. Vancomycin has to be infused over 1 hour to avoid hypotension and may increase inotrope requirement during surgery.

Careful surgical technique, haemostasis and use of the minimum amount of suture material are important in the reduction of the risk of infection. Excessive use of diathermy or sutures and prolonged opening and closure times are common risk factors. The obese patient, especially if diabetic, is most likely to develop infection because of the difficulty in opposing the wound edges and the prolonged surgical time.[24] After surgery, wound discharge in the early postoperative period is a major risk factor particularly if the wound dressing is changed prematurely or the wound is handled without adequate aseptic technique.

Key point 5

- MRSA is a major reason for litigation in surgery.

MEDICOLEGAL CONSEQUENCES OF MRSA

MRSA infections are well known to the public as hospital-associated and the media interest has been heightened by publication of hospital league tables of bacteraemia rates. The antibiotic resistance pattern of MRSA is often characteristic and can be used to infer the source of acquisition of an infection. There may be similar strains in other patients in the same ward or under the same surgeon.

MRSA is currently the most common cause of infection for which hospitals are sued. Most cases are settled out of Court, some for sums in excess of £1 million. Cases are often focused on the failure of staff to adhere to the control of infection policy through lack of hand hygiene or failure to screen or act on the result of screening when it was intended. Cases can be defended when hand hygiene and cleaning audits are available showing reasonable compliance and standards and documentation in the medical notes demonstrates reasonable care.

Key point 6

- Many wound infections develop in the ward due to contamination in the early postoperative period rather than from events in the theatre.

CONCLUSIONS

MRSA is now the major cause of nosocomial infection in many countries. Infection can be severe, prolonged and difficult to treat. Transmission of epidemic strains is wide-spread as the result of poor hand hygiene. Prolongation of hospital stay due to MRSA is a major cost pressure on hospitals. Prevention by means of screening, improvement of hand hygiene and good surgical technique is essential to reduce patient morbidity and improve surgical outcomes.

Key points for clinical practice

- MRSA infection increases mortality and length of hospital stay at least 3-fold.
- MRSA is more invasive and difficult to treat than other *Staphylococcus aureus* infections.
- MRSA is spread predominantly on the unwashed hands of staff.

(continued)

Key points for clinical practice *(continued)*

- Screening and topical decontamination reduces the risk of both MRSA infection in a patient and its spread to other patients.

- MRSA is a major reason for litigation in surgery.

- Many wound infections develop in the ward due to contamination in the early postoperative period rather than from events in the theatre.

References

1. Johnson AP, Pearson A, Duckworth G. Surveillance and epidemiology of MRSA bacteraemia in the UK. *J Antimicrob Chemother* 2005; **56**: 455–462.

2. Franchi D, Climo MW, Wong AH, Edmond MB, Wenzel RP. Seeking vancomycin resistant *Staphylococcus aureus* among patients with vancomycin-resistant enterococci. *Clin Infect Dis* 1999; **29**: 1566–1568.

3. Pujol M, Pena C, Pallares R *et al*. Nosocomial *Staphylococcus aureus* bacteremia among nasal carriers of methicillin-resistant and methicillin-susceptible strains. *Am J Med* 1996; **100**: 509–516.

4. Cosgrove SE, Qi Y, Kaye KS, Harbarth S, Karchmer AW, Carmeli Y. The impact of methicillin resistance in *Staphylococcus aureus* bacteremia on patient outcomes: mortality, length of stay, and hospital charges. *Infect Control Hosp Epidemiol* 2005; **26**: 166–174.

5. Romero-Vivas J, Rubio M, Fernandez C, Picazo JJ. Mortality associated with nosocomial bacteremia due to methicillin-resistant *Staphylococcus aureus*. *Clin Infect Dis* 1995; **21**: 1417–1423.

6. Watters K, O'Dwyer TP, Rowley H. Cost and morbidity of MRSA in head and neck cancer patients: what are the consequences? *J Laryngol Otol* 2004; **118**: 694–699.

7. Bagger JP, Zindrou D, Taylor KM. Postoperative infection with meticillin-resistant *Staphylococcus aureus* and socioeconomic background. *Lancet* 2004; **363**: 706–708.

8. Marshall C, Wolfe R, Kossmann T, Wesselingh S, Harrington G, Spelman D. Risk factors for acquisition of methicillin-resistant *Staphylococcus aureus* (MRSA) by trauma patients in the intensive care unit. *J Hosp Infect* 2004; **57**: 245–252.

9. Eckmanns T, Rath A, Brauer H, Daschner F, Ruden H, Gastmeier P. [Compliance with hand hygiene in intensive care units.] *Dtsch Med Wochenschr* 2001; **126**: 745–749.

10. MacDonald A, Dinah F, MacKenzie D, Wilson A. Performance feedback of hand hygiene, using alcohol gel as the skin decontaminant, reduces the number of inpatients newly affected by MRSA and antibiotic costs. *J Hosp Infect* 2004; **56**: 56–63.

11. Herr CE, Heckrodt TH, Hofmann FA, Schnettler R, Eikmann TF. Additional costs for preventing the spread of methicillin-resistant *Staphylococcus aureus* and a strategy for reducing these costs on a surgical ward. *Infect Control Hosp Epidemiol* 2003; **24**: 673–678.

12. Curran ET, Hamilton K, Monaghan A, McGinlay M, Thakker B. Use of a temporary cohort ward as part of an intervention to reduce the incidence of meticillin-resistant *Staphylococcus aureus* in a vascular surgery ward. *J Hosp Infect* 2006; **63**: 374–379.

13. Talon D, Vichard P, Muller A, Bertin M, Jeunet L, Bertrand X. Modelling the usefulness of a dedicated cohort facility to prevent the dissemination of MRSA. *J Hosp Infect* 2003; **54**: 57–62.

14. Cepeda JA, Whitehouse T, Cooper B *et al*. Isolation of patients in single rooms or cohorts to reduce spread of MRSA in intensive-care units: prospective two-centre study. *Lancet* 2005; **365**: 295–304.

15. Gemmell CG, Edwards DI, Fraise AP, Gould FK, Ridgway GL, Warren RE. Guidelines for the prophylaxis and treatment of methicillin-resistant *Staphylococcus aureus* (MRSA) infections in the UK. *J Antimicrob Chemother* 2006; **57**: 589–608.

16. Nixon M, Jackson B, Varghese P, Jenkins D, Taylor G. Methicillin-resistant *Staphylococcus aureus* on orthopaedic wards: incidence, spread, mortality, cost and control. *J Bone Joint Surg Br* 2006; **88**: 812–817.

17. Schelenz S, Tucker D, Georgeu C et al. Significant reduction of endemic MRSA acquisition and infection in cardiothoracic patients by means of an enhanced targeted infection control programme. *J Hosp Infect* 2005; **60**: 104–110.
18. Malde DJ, Abidia A, McCollum C, Welch M. The success of routine MRSA screening in vascular surgery: a nine year review. *Int Angiol* 2006; **25**: 204–208.
19. Loeb M, Main C, Walker-Dilks C, Eady A. Antimicrobial drugs for treating methicillin-resistant *Staphylococcus aureus* colonization. *Cochrane Database Syst Rev* 2003(4): CD003340.
20. Wilcox MH, Hall J, Pike H et al. Use of perioperative mupirocin to prevent methicillin-resistant *Staphylococcus aureus* (MRSA) orthopaedic surgical site infections. *J Hosp Infect* 2003; **54**: 196–201.
21. Suzuki Y, Kamigaki T, Fujino Y, Tominaga M, Ku Y, Kuroda Y. Randomized clinical trial of preoperative intranasal mupirocin to reduce surgical-site infection after digestive surgery. *Br J Surg* 2003; **90**: 1072–1075.
22. Wilson AP, Hodgson B, Liu M et al. Reduction in wound infection rates by wound surveillance with postdischarge follow-up and feedback. *Br J Surg* 2006; **93**: 630–638.
23. Merrer J, Pisica-Donose G, Leneveu M, Pauthier F. Prevalence of methicillin-resistant *Staphylococcus aureus* nasal carriage among patients with femoral neck fractures: implication for antibiotic prophylaxis. *Infect Control Hosp Epidemiol* 2004; **25**: 515–517.
24. Dodds Ashley ES, Carroll DN, Engemann JJ et al. Risk factors for postoperative mediastinitis due to methicillin-resistant Staphylococcus aureus. *Clin Infect Dis* 2004; **38**: 1555–1560.

Sandip Sarkar   Alexander M. Seifalian

3

Tissue engineering of blood vessels

The recent successful clinical application of tissue-engineered bladders[1] has moved the topic of tissue-engineered blood vessels from the realms of science fiction into the forefront of the public imagination, due to the realisation that more complex organ-engineering may be feasible, but only with integrated vascular networks to nourish the various tissue planes. In fact, the development of tissue-engineered vascular bypass grafts has been a thriving research field for the last 20 years, with particular emphasis on small calibre (< 6 mm) cardiovascular bypass conduits. This is driven by the dismal long-term patency of expanded polytetrafluoroethylene (ePTFE) grafts used in distal infra-inguinal bypass[2] (less than 30% at 5 years) and the considerable proportion (30%) of patients in whom the preferred alternative (long saphenous vein) is unavailable.[3] With the ageing population comes an increasing incidence of re-operation for distal peripheral vascular disease or previous coronary bypass where the saphenous vein has already been harvested. The poor result with synthetic materials is due to the large number of diverse functions which are asked of graft materials, and are ably provided by arteries. Hence, the ability to engineer an artery to order is an attractive proposition. Furthermore, it also opens up a whole field of paediatric vascular surgery, eliminating the need for sequential replacement of synthetic grafts in paediatric patients.[4]

Sandip Sarkar MA MRCS (Glasg)
Vascular Research Fellow. Academic Division of Surgical & Interventional Sciences, University College London, Rowland Hill Street, London NW3 2PF, UK

Alexander M. Seifalian PhD FInstNano (for correspondence)
Professor, Academic Division of Surgical & Interventional Sciences, University College London, Rowland Hill Street, London NW3 2PF, UK
E-mail: a.seifalian@medsch.ucl.ac.uk

21

Key point 1

- The greatest need for a tissue engineered vascular graft is in bypass of small diameter (< 6 mm) arteries.

IDEAL GRAFT CHARACTERISTICS

Table 1 shows the ideal vascular bypass prosthesis specification. Traditional synthetic material technologies have not been able to provide for all of these criteria simultaneously. This inability to suit purpose completely is particularly critical in the low-flow states observed in vessels smaller than 6 mm.

High-flow environments allow compromise of arterial properties, as is shown in the excellent results of knitted Dacron® (polyethylene terephthalate) as an aortic graft. Current synthetic grafts fulfil few of the standards, but have the significant advantage over tissue-engineered vessels of being mass-producible on an industrial scale, making them readily available in a variety of dimensions.

Table 1 The ideal vascular bypass graft specification

Parameters	Essential	Desirable
Mechanical properties	Mechanical strength to withstand physiological haemodynamic pressure	Compliance matching with native artery
		Modulation of mechanical properties depending on changes in haemodynamics in short and long term
Blood compatibility	Low thrombogenicity	Non-thrombogenic
		Localised coagulation at site of injury to vessel wall
Biocompatibility	Long-term biostability	Good graft healing and endothelialisation without excessive fibrovascular infiltration compromising vessel calibre and compliance
	Non-immunogenic	
Functional properties		Incorporation of homeostatic/ regulatory mechanisms, e.g. nitric oxide, prostacyclin release
		Infection resistance
Availability	Available quickly in urgent cases	Available without further invasive procedures for the patient

COMPONENTS REQUIRED FOR TISSUE-ENGINEERED VASCULAR GRAFTS

An artery meets all the requirements for haemodynamic propulsion via a composite structure with different elements concentrating on different properties as well as a keen interaction on a structural and biomolecular level. Figure 1 shows a diagrammatic representation of the layered arterial wall structure.

Key point 2

- Tissue engineering aims to replicate the structural and cellular organisation of an artery to confer the diverse range of properties necessary for arterial function.

Many approaches have been used to achieve the common goal of viable confluent sheets of cells anchored on a tubular scaffold. The role of the scaffold is to provide shape as well as initial strength. Some investigators have done away with the need for a scaffold altogether, using a mandrel on which cellular attachment, adherence and confluence are encouraged using cell culture techniques in a bioreactor (Fig. 2).[5] However, the use of a matrix or scaffold into which cells can embed are generally more successful.[6] The scaffolds used

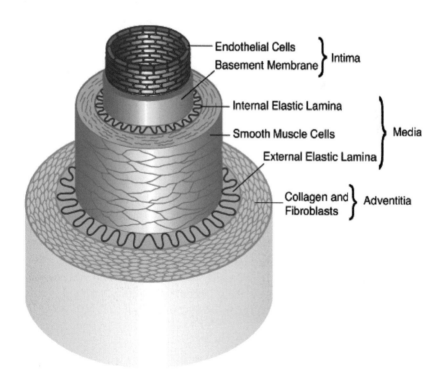

Endothelial Cells
Basement Membrane } Intima

Internal Elastic Lamina
Smooth Muscle Cells } Media
External Elastic Lamina

Collagen and
Fibroblasts } Adventitia

Fig. 1 The multiple laminar organisation of the arterial wall allows it to maintain a wide range of properties.

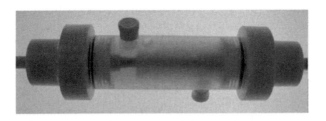

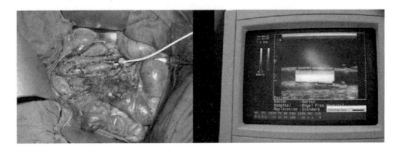

Fig. 2 A living cellular matrix, comprising of Type I collagen and porcine smooth muscle cells, which is contracted on a central mandrel within a bioreactor and after endothelisation being evaluated *in vivo* using a porcine infrarenal aortic model.

are either synthetic or biologically sourced. In the case of the former, a non-degrading material will result in a hybrid graft rather than a wholly tissue-engineered graft and their mechanical properties will reflect those of the scaffold, with limited capacity for adaptation to changing blood flow conditions. Few such scaffolds have resulted in a clinically successful bypass graft.[7] These will not be considered further as the permanent presence of the scaffold compromises the ultimate aim of replication of true arterial function. Biodegradable scaffolds have been shown to provide a suitable environment for adherence, proliferation and organisation of cells. They provide primary mechanical stability while the cellular structures mature. As demonstrated in Figure 3, the scaffold initially withstands the stresses of pulsatile flow. As the scaffold begins to degrade and formation of matrix occurs, the newly regenerating cells are gradually loaded with physiological stress, further simulating tissue regeneration. Eventually, the scaffold completely degrades and the regenerated tissue bears the stress. Biological scaffolds may be transplanted tissues or specifically constructed, using extracellular matrix components. The cells in consideration are fibroblasts, smooth muscle cells (SMCs) and vascular endothelial cells (ECs; Fig. 3). The attachment of progenitor stem cells is an exciting recent possibility,[8] aimed at rapid accumulation of appropriate cellular layers, including cell adherence from endogenous blood flow.

MECHANICAL PROPERTIES

Mechanical characterisation of the artery reveals an anisotropic nature with high elasticity at low pressures and greater stiffness along with low

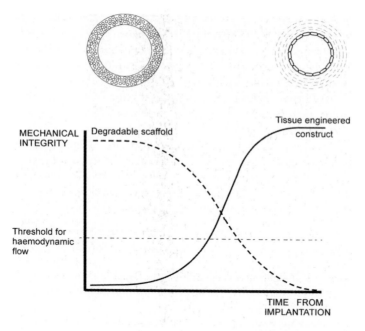

Fig. 3 The time-line for the development of a tissue-engineered bypass graft using a synthetic biodegradable scaffold, which is gradually replaced by arterial matrix with an endothelial lining. Concept for diagram modified from Berglund et al.[9]

distensibility at high pressures.[2] This is due to the multilaminar arrangement of collagen and elastin with the former providing high tensile strength as individual fibres are gradually recruited at increasing pressures, and the latter accounting for high distensibility (Fig. 1). The combination of strength and elasticity has been a particular challenge in potential synthetic graft development, with modification of traditional materials such as segmented polyurethanes allowing an improvement in one at the expense of the other by modification of the soft and hard segments. It is felt that the inequality of elasticity (compliance mismatch) between native artery and graft material may be responsible for intimal hyperplasia, which itself is the cause of medium to long-term graft occlusion of small calibre grafts. It is essential, therefore, to consider an appropriate extracellular matrix (ECM) for tissue engineering grafts to mirror the strength and elasticity of arteries.

One principle by which to achieve this aim is to use a biodegradable hydrophilic polymer scaffold, with long-term replacement by ECM. The bioresorbable scaffolds used are based on polyglycolic acid (PGA), polydioxanone or polylactide. PGA forms a porous structure but is resorbed within 8 weeks; in order to slow degradation, it is often combined with an adjunct such as polyhydroxyalkanoate, poly-4-hydroxybutyrate or polyethylene glycol.[10] Cellular infiltration of these scaffolds is dependent on a highly porous, open structure.

Many groups have considered collagen itself as the foundation for biological scaffolds, primarily because of the impressive strength it imparts. However, Weinberg and Bell's pioneering collagen-based scaffolds were very weak, requiring a Dacron mesh for initial strength.[11] Berglund et al.[12] have shown that elastin makes collagen tubes stronger – it may have a considerable role in distributing the stress across the tissue-engineered vessel wall. Elastin also improves the viscous nature which again is generally thought to be due to collagen. Without elastin's gradual stretching influence, the abrupt pressure wave on the collagen construct may not allow sufficient time for the viscous component to manifest itself. Berglund and colleagues extracted elastin scaffolds from an animal model by targeted enzymatic digestion of ECM. However, it is very difficult to incorporate elastin into engineered structures due to its low solubility. Leach's group[13] have used water-soluble α-elastin in conjunction with a 'molecular glue' to form 'elastin-like' structures with similar mechanical and cell-adherent properties. An added advantage is that the materials used are readily available off the shelf.

Key point 3

- In order to achieve arterial visco-elasticity as well as strength, both collagen and elastin properties need to be represented.

Collagen also derives strength from circumferentially arranged SMC layers which require prolonged culture to achieve as well as a porous collagen network. The orientation of the SMC is paramount and can be optimised by pulsatile flow in bioreactors which cause circumferential stress as a stimulus.[14]

Polymeric mandrels, when placed subcutaneously or intraperitoneally, cause a fibrous foreign-body reaction, effectively coating the mandrel with a strong collagenous tube which can be used as a scaffold.[15] Physiological flow on implantation results in further collagen thickening, elastin deposition and myofibroblastic re-organisation.

Other derivatives of biological structures which may act as temporary scaffolds, to be replaced by ECM are gaining prominence. The work of Lepidi et al.[16] on hyaluronan (an esterified hyaluronate) is promising, showing rapid accumulation of organised arterial cellular and ECM components in an animal model, with biodegradation of the scaffold over 4 months. The cellular re-organisation is undoubtedly helped by the scaffold's ability to maintain a loosely packed ECM. However, this success in microvessels has yet to be shown in their 3–6 mm counterparts as the strength of the construct is strongly dependent on the ECM formed.[17]

Key point 4

- The use of modified derivatives of biological materials to form scaffolds is gaining prominence due to the ease of obtaining and handling these raw materials as well as their propensity to encourage formal vascular extracellular matrix formation.

BLOOD COMPATIBILITY

It is notoriously difficult to render a synthetic material non-thrombogenic, requiring the concomitant properties of hydrophilicity, electronegativity and inertness. Currently, the best hope is for the development of an endothelial lining. This is not due to a physical smooth surface presented by the endothelial layer – rather it is due to the mechanisms of coagulation regulation incorporated into each endothelial cell as well as an efficient intracellular signalling system triggered by the prevailing haemodynamic conditions. In addition, it is a physical barrier separating blood from the moderately thrombogenic basement membrane and the highly thrombogenic collagen of the ECM. Unfortunately, although some animal models readily endothelialise,[18] a synthetic graft with long confluent endothelialised sections in clinical practice is yet to be achieved. Recognising this, some groups have accepted the need for blood interaction with collagen, turning to surface modifications of collagen such as heparin-bonding which can be partially successful in reducing thrombogenicity.[19]

Key point 5

- A confluent endothelial lining is critically important in a tissue-engineered graft to prevent thrombosis.

Tissue engineering aims to provide low graft thrombogenicity via active seeding of the blood interface with ECs. Careful consideration must be given to the source of EC along with the method of extraction and seeding. Most recently, the possibility of recruiting endothelial progenitor cells (EPCs) circulating in the blood, which subsequently differentiate into endothelial cells, is being realised *in vitro*, as is the seeding of pluripotent stem cells from bone marrow and adipose tissue.

SOURCES OF ENDOTHELIAL CELLS

VEINS

Although endothelial cell extraction has been successfully performed from the vein wall, optimal seeding and culture on synthetic scaffolds requires a turn-over time of at least 7 days.[20] However, the degree of adherence and function of the seeded cells depends greatly on the scaffold material used. This is perfectly illustrated by Yeh and colleagues' study of endothelial cells seeded to different metallic stent materials,[21] showing the importance of considering not only attachment but also the level of function for these cells.

Key point 6

- The good patency of saphenous vein grafts mean that tissue-engineered vascular grafts need not be considered for distal infra-inguinal bypass if saphenous vein is available.

Of course it can be argued that using available vein as graft material is already successful in the case of small-calibre vessel bypass, eliminating the need for tissue-engineering in these cases.

ADIPOSE

Oedayrajsingh-Varma et al.[22] have shown that adipose-derived stem cells with true proliferative potential could be harvested with greater efficiency from surgically excised adipose tissue than from ultrasound-guided liposuction. However, these cells differentiated into connective tissue rather than endothelial cells and it is not clear whether the same would apply for endothelial progenitors. In fact, it is becoming evident that the differentiation potential for these adipose-derived stem cells may include several different lineages, dependent on biomolecular environmental cues rather than it being genetically predetermined.[23,24] Endothelial progenitor cells can differentiate into SMCs under certain conditions, but they are unable to proliferate themselves.

BONE MARROW

This is a ready source of pluripotent stem cells, which will be available at the time of surgery. Cho and colleagues[25] seeded small-calibre decellularised canine carotids with ECs and SMCs of bone marrow origin before implantation and found 8-week patency as well as a regenerated arterial wall. However, these cells were cultured *in vitro* for 3 weeks meaning that bone marrow biopsy was required separately to operation. Shin'oka's group[26] have demonstrated endothelium-like cells on biodegrading scaffolds after fixing unselected bone marrow cells with fibrin glue and a maturation time of only 4 hours.

BIOSTABILITY

The tissue-engineered graft is continually moulded depending on the haemodynamic demands placed on it.[27] So it may be seen that the original ECM scaffolds used are not recognisable after being implanted for some time. However, as with synthetic grafts, ECM scaffolds are vulnerable to unintended biodegradation, leading to graft-wall weakness, aneurysm and failure. This is a particular problem with elastin in decellularised xenograft scaffolds, which degrades despite gluteraldehyde-fixation due to its low opportunities for cross-linking. Tannic acid is commonly used as a fixative for elastin before electron microscopy, and this can be used to prevent its biodegradation by forming cross-linking hydrogen bonds between hydrophobic regions of the chain.[28]

Key point 7

- Tissue-engineered scaffolds may be susceptible to biodegradation despite being manufactured from the same components found in arterial extracellular matrix.

OFF-THE-SHELF AVAILABILITY

Arterial bypass grafts are required on a semi-urgent basis for the relief of critical ischaemia and, in some cases, urgently after the onset of acute ischaemia which may occur after interventional radiological procedures have been attempted. One great criticism levelled at tissue-engineering grafts is the long-time period required before an individualised graft can be made available. Attempts to use readily available ECM components are being made and this has been discussed with respect to elastin above.[13,16] Collagen hydrogels are convenient for forming scaffolds, although they may be shrunk by the developing confluent cell layers. Lewus and Nauman[29] have determined that this undesirable effect is reduced by including whole collagen fibres to the hydrogel matrix.

Much of the time presently required for cell seeding is attributable to the two-stage procedure of cell culture followed by seeding in a bioreactor. Niklason's group[30] have demonstrated a direct correlation between the time for maturation and strength of the resultant graft.

To address this, a single-stage method aimed at simplifying and quickening the graft implantation process involves autoseeding cells rather than relying on physical extraction of cells by enzymatic or physical means where cell yields are low and adhesive efficiency and then proliferation is limited. This latter yields different levels of differentiation of SMC lines depending on the method of extraction.[31]

Some biodegradable synthetic polymers have relatively poor cell adherence properties, making them very unlikely to autoseed from peripheral blood. Binding these materials with collagen may enhance their cellularisation capability greatly,[32,33] leading to the possibility of autoseeding.

An alternative prospect for autoseeding is EPCs which have been shown to circulate in peripheral blood, and could contribute to rapid endothelialisation of scaffolds.[34] Work on animal models in this area must be interpreted with a degree of caution as endothelialisation occurs less readily in humans. Also, the number of circulating EPCs in whole blood is low and the time taken for confluent endothelialisation by autoseeding without cell culture is high. Notwithstanding this, Shirota's department has shown effective endothelialisation with human EPCs on collagen-coated polyurethane conduits.[35] The problem of low EPC numbers in circulating blood can be circumvented by rapid seeding of stem cell-rich bone marrow as discussed previously. Another alternative may be to persuade the bone marrow to mobilise larger numbers of EPCs, using granulocyte colony stimulating factor and granulocyte-macrophage colony stimulating factor.[36]

Other mechanisms to improve endothelialisation efficiency include surface modifications with RGD-containing peptides[37] and growth factors such as basic fibroblast growth factor.[38] The RGD moiety is also independently antithrombogenic[39] and increases the feasibility of a single-stage seeding procedure.[40]

Key point 8

- Clinical applicability of tissue-engineered grafts is greatly dependent on the time-scale required for graft preparation as well as the acceptability of the method for preparation.

To date, there is only one group that has used the principles of vascular tissue engineering clinically. Shin'oka and colleagues[41] seeded a biodegrading scaffold and used the resultant tissue as a pulmonary artery graft in a child. Similarly, they have also demonstrated the use of tissue engineered tissue (both using SMCs and bone marrow derived stem cells) for pulmonary arterial and venous congenital anomaly surgery.[4,26] It is perhaps not surprising that the only clinical reports relate to paediatric surgery as the current alternative is repeated major surgical procedures using synthetic materials which need replacing as the child grows. However, these cases all relate to low haemodynamic pressure systems.

The major clinical use of a tissue-engineered vascular graft will involve long-term implantation in critical small vessel arterial systems such as the coronary circulation with exposure to systemic blood pressures. This will require extensive testing *in vivo*, including higher species and subsequent primate implantation before formal clinical trials. Unfortunately, much of the established *in vivo* work is in small animals, with high trans-anastomotic endothelialisation rates which do not mirror graft behaviour in humans.

Key point 9

- Long-standing in vivo study in appropriate animal models will be required before tissue-engineered grafts can enter wide-spread clinical use.

Key points for clinical practice

- The greatest need for a tissue engineered vascular graft is in bypass of small diameter (< 6 mm) arteries.

- Tissue engineering aims to replicate the structural and cellular organisation of an artery to confer the diverse range of properties necessary for arterial function.

- In order to achieve arterial visco-elasticity as well as strength, both collagen and elastin properties need to be represented.

- The use of modified derivatives of biological materials to form scaffolds is gaining prominence due to the ease of obtaining and handling these raw materials as well as their propensity to encourage formal vascular extracellular matrix formation.

- A confluent endothelial lining is critically important in a tissue-engineered graft to prevent thrombosis.

- The good patency of saphenous vein grafts mean that tissue-engineered vascular grafts need not be considered for distal infra-inguinal bypass if saphenous vein is available.

- Tissue-engineered scaffolds may be susceptible to biodegradation despite being manufactured from the same components found in arterial extracellular matrix. *(continued)*

Key points for clinical practice *(continued)*

- Clinical applicability of tissue-engineered grafts is greatly dependent on the time-scale required for graft preparation as well as the acceptability of the method for preparation.

- Long-standing in vivo study in appropriate animal models will be required before tissue-engineered grafts can enter wide-spread

References

1. Atala A, Bauer SB, Soker S, Yoo JJ, Retik AB. Tissue-engineered autologous bladders for patients needing cystoplasty. *Lancet* 2006; **367**: 1241–1246.
2. Sarkar S, Salacinski HJ, Hamilton G, Seifalian AM. The mechanical properties of infrainguinal vascular bypass grafts: their role in influencing patency. *Eur J Vasc Endovasc Surg* 2006; **31**: 627–636.
3. Veith FJ, Moss CM, Sprayregen S. Preoperative saphenous venography in arterial reconstructive surgery of the lower extremity. *Surgery* 1979; **85**: 253–256.
4. Matsumura G, Hibino N, Ikada Y, Kurosawa H, Shin'oka T. Successful application of tissue engineered vascular autografts: clinical experience. *Biomaterials* 2003; **24**: 2303–2308.
5. Baguneid MS, Siefalian AM, Hamilton G, Walker MG. Development of a tissue-engineered small-diameter vascular graft. *Br J Surg* 2000; **87**: 87.
6. Abilez O, Benharash P, Mehrotra M *et al.* A novel culture system shows that stem cells can be grown in 3D and under physiological pulsatile conditions for tissue engineering of vascular grafts. *J Surg Res* 2006; **132**: 170–178.
7. Zilla P, Deutsch M, Meinhart J. Endothelial cell transplantation. *Semin Vasc Surg* 1999; **12**: 52–63.
8. Riha GM, Lin PH, Lumsden AB, Yao Q, Chen C. Application of stem cells for vascular tissue engineering. *Tissue Eng* 2005; 11: 1535–1552.
9. Berglund JD, Mohseni MM, Nerem RM, Sambanis A. A biological hybrid model for collagen-based tissue engineered vascular constructs. *Biomaterials* 2003; **24**: 1241–1254.
10. Kakisis JD, Liapis CD, Breuer C, Sumpio BE. Artificial blood vessel: the Holy Grail of peripheral vascular surgery. *J Vasc Surg* 2005; **41**: 349–354.
11. Weinberg CB, Bell E. A blood vessel model constructed from collagen and cultured vascular cells. *Science* 1986; **231**: 397–400.
12. Berglund JD, Nerem RM, Sambanis A. Incorporation of intact elastin scaffolds in tissue-engineered collagen-based vascular grafts. *Tissue Eng* 2004; **10**: 1526–1535.
13. Leach JB, Wolinsky JB, Stone PJ, Wong JY. Crosslinked alpha-elastin biomaterials: towards a processable elastin-mimetic scaffold. *Acta Biomater* 2005; **1**: 155–164.
14. L'Heureux N, Germain L, Labbe R, Auger FA. *In vitro* construction of a human blood vessel from cultured vascular cells: a morphologic study. *J Vasc Surg* 1993; **17**: 499–509.
15. Nakayama Y, Ishibashi-Ueda H, Takamizawa K. *In vivo* tissue-engineered small-caliber arterial graft prosthesis consisting of autologous tissue (biotube). *Cell Transplant* 2004; **13**: 439–449.
16. Lepidi S, Abatangelo G, Vindigni V *et al. In vivo* regeneration of small-diameter (2 mm) arteries using a polymer scaffold. *FASEB J* 2006; **20**: 103–105.
17. Remuzzi A, Mantero S, Columbo M *et al.* Vascular smooth muscle cells on hyaluronic acid: culture and mechanical characterization of an engineered vascular construct. *Tissue Eng* 2004; **10**: 699–710.
18. Rashid ST, Salacinski HJ, Hamilton G, Seifalian AM. The use of animal models in developing the discipline of cardiovascular tissue engineering: a review. *Biomaterials* 2004; **25**: 1627–1637.
19. Keuren JF, Wielders SJ, Driessen A, Verhoeven M, Hendriks M, Lindhout T. Covalently bound heparin makes collagen thromboresistant. *Arterioscler Thromb Vasc Biol* 2004; **24**: 613–617.

20. Hsu SH, Tsai IJ, Lin DJ, Chen DC. The effect of dynamic culture conditions on endothelial cell seeding and retention on small diameterpolyurethane vascular grafts. *Med Eng Phys* 2005; **27**: 267–272.
21. Yeh H-I, Lu S-K, Tian T-Y, Hong R-C, Lee W-H, Tsai C-H. Comparison of endothelial cells grown on different stent materials. *J Biomed Mater Res A* 2006; **76**: 835–841.
22. Oedayrajsingh-Varma MJ, van Ham SM, Knippenberg M *et al*. Adipose tissue-derived mesenchymal stem cell yield and growth characteristics are affected by the tissue-harvesting procedure. *Cytotherapy* 2006; **8**: 166–177.
23. Nakagami H, Morishita R, Maeda K, Kikuchi Y, Ogihara T, Kaneda Y. Adipose tissue-derived stromal cells as a novel option for regenerative cell therapy. *J Atheroscler Thromb* 2006; **13**: 77–81.
24. Noer A, Sorensen AL, Boquest AC, Collas P. Stable CpG hypomethylation of adipogenic promoters in freshly isolated, cultured and differentiated mesenchymal stem cells from adipose tissue. *Mol Biol Cell* 2006; **17**: 3543–3556.
25. Cho SW, Lim SH, Kim IK *et al*. Small-diameter blood vessels engineered with bone marrow-derived cells. *Ann Surg* 2005; **241**: 506–515.
26. Shin'oka T, Matsumura G, Hibino N *et al*. Midterm clinical result of tissue-engineered vascular autografts seeded with autologous bone marrow cells. *J Thorac Cardiovasc Surg* 2005; **129**: 1330–1338.
27. Niklason LE, Gao J, Abbott WM *et al*. Functional arteries grown *in vitro*. *Science* 1999; **284**: 489–493.
28. Isenburg JC, Simionescu DT, Vyavahare NR. Elastin stabilization in cardiovascular implants: improved resistance to enzymatic degradation by treatment with tannic acid. *Biomaterials* 2004; **25**: 3293–3302.
29. Lewus KE, Nauman EA. *In vitro* characterization of a bone marrow stem cell-seeded collagen gel composite for soft tissue grafts: effects of fiber number and serum concentration. *Tissue Eng* 2005; **11**: 1015–1022.
30. Niklason LE, Abbott WM, Gao J *et al*. Morphologic and mechanical characteristics of engineered bovine arteries. *J Vasc Surg* 2001; **33**: 628–638.
31. Opitz F, Schenke-Layland K, Richter W *et al*. Tissue engineering of ovine aortic blood vessel substitutes using applied shear stress and enzymatically derived vascular smooth muscle cells. *Ann Biomed Eng* 2004; **32**: 212–222.
32. Ma Z, He W, Yong T, Ramakrishna S. Grafting of gelatin on electrospun poly(caprolactone) nanofibers to improve endothelial cell spreading and proliferation and to control cell orientation. *Tissue Eng* 2005; **11**: 1149–1158.
33. Iwai S, Sawa Y, Ichikawa H *et al*. Biodegradable polymer with collagen microsponge serves as a new bioengineered cardiovascular prosthesis. *J Thorac Cardiovasc Surg* 2004; **128**: 472–479.
34. He H, Shirota T, Yasui H, Matsuda T. Canine endothelial progenitor cell-lined hybrid vascular graft with nonthrombogenic potential. *J Thorac Cardiovasc Surg* 2003; **126**: 455–464.
35. Shirota T, He H, Yasui H, Matsuda H. Human endothelial progenitor cell-seeded hybrid graft: proliferative and antithrombogenic potentials *in vitro* and fabrication processing. *Tissue Eng* 2003; **9**: 127–136.
36. Cho SW, Lim JE, Chu HS *et al*. Enhancement of *in vivo* endothelialization of tissue-engineered vascular grafts by granulocyte colony-stimulating factor. *J Biomed Mater Res A* 2006; **76**: 252–263.
37. Hsu SH, Sun SH, Chen DC. Improved retention of endothelial cells seeded on polyurethane small-diameter vascular grafts modified by a recombinant RGD-containing protein. *Artif Organs* 2003; **27**: 1068–1078.
38. Conklin BS, Wu H, Lin PH, Lumsden AB, Chen C. Basic fibroblast growth factor coating and endothelial cell seeding of a decellularized heparin-coated vascular graft. *Artif Organs* 2004; **28**: 668–675.
39. Eriksson AC, Whiss PA. Measurement of adhesion of human platelets in plasma to protein surfaces in microplates. *J Pharmacol Toxicol Methods* 2005; **52**: 356–365.
40. Tiwari A, Kidane A, Salacinski HJ, Punshon G, Hamilton G, Siefalian AM. Improving endothelial cell retention for single stage seeding of prosthetic grafts: use of polymer sequences of arginine-glycine-aspartate. *Eur J Vasc Endovasc Surg* 2003; **25**: 325–329.
41. Shin'oka T, Imai Y, Ikada Y. Transplantation of a tissue-engineered pulmonary artery. *N Engl J Med* 2001; **344**: 532–533.

Douglas McWhinnie Ian Jackson

Newer procedures for day surgery

In the UK, day surgery is defined as 'the admission of selected patients to hospital for a planned surgical procedure, returning home on the same day'.[1] Any patient who remains in hospital at midnight is classified as an 'in-patient' as they have since the founding of the NHS in 1948. The day-surgery literature can be confusing as the term 'day surgery' is sometimes applied to an overnight stay (23 hours), especially in North America. Thus, when evaluating ambulatory data, it is important to ensure that definitions are consistent. The other major criticism of day surgery data is that there is little level 3 evidence (randomised control trials) comparing day surgery to in-patient outcomes. Day surgery, however, is a process, not a procedure. When measured outcomes relate to the patient pathway, rather than the surgical end result, then the advantages of day surgery are apparent.

BENCHMARKING

Day-surgery rates in the UK are based on the Audit Commission 'Basket of Procedures' last updated in the year 2001.[2] The 'basket' comprises 25 procedures across the surgical specialities and represents those operations most commonly performed on a day-case basis (Table 1). These data are, therefore, useful in benchmarking day-surgery activity between health authorities, hospital trusts and even individual surgeons. The downside of such a benchmarking tool is that it becomes rapidly out of date. With the

Douglas McWhinnie MD FRCS (for correspondence)
Clinical Lead for Day Surgery, Consultant General Surgeon, Milton Keynes General Hospital NHS Trust, Standing Way, Eaglestone MK6 5LD, UK
E-mail: douglas.mcwhinnie@mkgeneral.nhs.uk

Ian Jackson MMB ChB(Aberdeen) FRCA
Clinical Lead for Day Surgery, Consultant Anaesthetist, York Hospitals NHS Trust, York YO30 8HE, UK

Table 1 Audit Commission basket of 25 procedures 2001

- Orchidopexy
- Circumcision
- Inguinal hernia repair
- Excision of breast lump
- Anal fissure dilatation
- Haemorrhoidectomy
- Laparoscopic cholecystectomy
- Varicose vein stripping or ligation
- Transurethral resection of bladder tumour
- Excision of Dupuytren's contracture
- Carpal tunnel decompression
- Excision of ganglion
- Arthroscopy
- Bunion operations
- Removal of metalware
- Extraction of cataract with or without implant
- Correction of squint
- Myringotomy
- Tonsillectomy
- Submucous resection
- Reduction of nasal fracture
- Operation for bat ears
- Dilatation and curettage/hysteroscopy
- Laparoscopy
- Termination of pregnancy

current rationalisation of hospital services, only 12% of trusts perform 75% or more of the 'basket'.[3]

Recently introduced procedures in day surgery are omitted while existing 'basket' procedures may be less frequently performed as new technology, techniques or overt rationing renders the procedure non-representative of current day-surgery activity. For example, out-patient hysteroscopy has largely replaced dilatation and curettage, MRI scanning has reduced the need for diagnostic arthroscopy and rationing of 'non-essential' varicose vein surgery by many PCTs has reduced the number of vein patients suitable for day surgery as severe varicose eczema or ulceration is more likely in the older, less fit patient.

Published basket day-case rates vary by region throughout the UK. Currently, the national average for England is 69.8%,[4] which is still far short of the 75% target published in the NHS Plan[5] which was to have been achieved by April 2005. Indeed, over the past 5 years, the increase in day-surgery activity has been about 1% per annum. Comparable day surgery rates in Scotland (56%), and Wales (60%) remain lower than in England.[6,7] Data for Northern Ireland is not comparable as the benchmarking basket of procedures is not equivalent. Despite the prominence given to achieving high day-case rates and their associated potential savings in in-patient bed-days, major fiscal benefit can be delivered by reducing the overall length of stay for elective surgical procedures. The application of day-surgery principles (pre-assessment, day of surgery admission and protocol-driven discharge) to the short-stay pathway offers substantial bed-day savings when applied to high-volume procedures and encourages a procedure shift from in-patient to 23-hour stay, 23-hour stay to day case and day case to out-patients or primary care. This shift is reflected in the British Association of Day Surgery directory of 160 procedures where aspirational percentages for each of these management options are offered.[8] It allows newer day-surgery or potential day-surgery procedures to be evaluated at an early stage, and provides a useful benchmarking tool not simply for day surgery but for the entire short-stay pathway.

Key point 1–3

- The NHS Plan indicated that the day surgery target should be 75% of the Audit Commission 'basket' of 25 procedures.

- Day-surgery rates remain lower than expected with the average for England (69.8%), Wales (60%) and Scotland (50%) all below 75%.

- The British Association of Day Surgery directory offers aspirational percentages for 160 short-stay procedures as out-patient procedures, day cases, 23-hour cases, short-stay cases (< 72 hours).

DEVELOPMENT OF DAY-SURGERY PROCEDURES

In determining whether a procedure is suitable to be performed on a day-case basis, certain criteria must be considered. The duration of the procedure should be less than 2 hours, postoperative pain must be easily controlled and any serious or life-threatening complications would have happened regardless of keeping the patient overnight. It is the patient and not the operation which is ambulatory; in embarking upon newer procedures for day surgery, careful patient selection with appropriate pre-operative assessment is essential.

The growth of day surgery over the past decade is the result of developments in anaesthesia and analgesia, as well as the surgery itself. Newer short-acting anaesthetic agents have been produced with minimal side-effects. Laryngeal mask anaesthesia negates the need for endotracheal intubation and pre-emptive and multimodal analgesia offers good control of peri-operative pain.

Surgical developments include the introduction of minimal access surgery for traditional procedures, new techniques offering alternative methods of operation and the revisiting of traditional surgical procedures on a day-case basis as a result of longer duration of anaesthesia.

Key point 4

- Day-surgery developments are the result of improvements in anaesthesia and analgesia as well as the surgery itself.

ANAESTHESIA AND ANALGESIA

Success in day surgery is dependent on a team and an important member is the anaesthetist. Managing more challenging patients and those undergoing more complex procedures requires meticulous technique to minimise postoperative problems such as pain, nausea and vomiting, dizziness and sore throat. Indeed, the Association of Anaesthetists states: 'Each anaesthetist should develop techniques that permit the patient to undergo the surgical procedure with minimum stress, maximum comfort and optimise their chance of early discharge'.[9]

Sadly, this requirement is neglected in many units and this leads to an increased unplanned admission rate. Modern anaesthetic agents such as Desflurane and Sevoflurane are ideally suited to day surgery as is total intravenous anaesthesia (TIVA) with Propofol. There is no one 'ideal' anaesthetic agent or technique but there are many common principles.

Key point 5

- Newer procedures for day surgery occur as a result of the introduction of new technologies and techniques, or revisiting traditional surgical procedures due to safer, extended-duration anaesthesia.

Education of the patient and their carer

This should start at the Pre-operative Assessment Clinic with both verbal and written information. Staff involved should have a good knowledge of the procedure being discussed so that the patient does not receive conflicting advice.

Drugs prior to surgery

Non-steroidal anti-inflammatory drugs (NSAIDs) should be given whenever there are no contra-indications. The use of intravenous or PR routes of administration is not necessary and there is evidence that giving the first dose orally about 1 hour pre-operatively produces better and longer lasting pain relief.[10]

Paracetamol may also be given pre-operatively, by the oral route reducing the need for more potent opioids with their unwanted side-effects. However, intravenous paracetamol is now available in the UK, is fast acting and appears more effective than oral paracetamol with analgesic effects comparable to NSAIDs.

Intra-operative technique

Infiltrating with local anaesthesia prior to making any skin incision reduces the amount of anaesthetic required by the patient and reduces postoperative pain more than infiltration at the end of a procedure. There is no evidence to support the routine use of prophylactic anti-emetics for every day-case patient, but these should form part of the anaesthetic protocol for specific procedures *e.g.* laparoscopic cholecystectomy and bariatric surgery. Long-acting opioids (and morphine in particular) increase the incidence of postoperative nausea and vomiting (PONV) even in small doses but, if used carefully, does not necessarily prevent scheduled discharge.[11] The use of intravenous fluids has been shown to reduce the incidence of thirst, drowsiness and dizziness[12] and may also benefit PONV.

Recovery

Where possible, beds should be avoided. Many units are now successfully using recliner chairs at an early stage of the recovery process and find this helps the mobilisation of the patient.

Oral analgesics remain the mainstay of pain control following day surgery. NSAIDs in association with paracetamol/codeine combination tablets are the most commonly prescribed analgesics in day surgery.[13] As larger operations are undertaken, day-case units are looking at the use of Oramorph or newer agents such as Oxycodone as discharge drugs. Whichever drug is prescribed, it is important that the patient receives the first dose prior to discharge and before the effect of any short-acting opioids or local anaesthesia wears off. With larger operations, the patient should also be advised about the requirement for regular dosing for the first few days to avoid 'breakthrough pain'.

NEWER DAY-SURGERY PROCEDURES

Anti-reflux surgery

Laparoscopic Nissen fundiplication for gastro-oesophageal reflux disease as a day case is gaining popularity. The main barrier to discharge is prolonged operating time beyond 2 hours. Thus, a skilled and experienced laparoscopist is essential to ensure success. Day-case surgery rates of 80% in 113 anti-reflux procedures have been reported[14] with high rates (95%) of favourable patient response.[15] Unrecognised mucosal perforation remains a concern but, even with an overnight stay, such complications may not always be recognised before discharge.

Bariatric surgery

Surgery for morbid obesity (body mass index > 40 kg/m^2) is on the increase as the financial and human cost of sickness and premature death is recognised. The problems with day-case laparoscopic gastric banding include the technical surgical problems of operating on the obese abdomen and the anaesthetic complications of airway control, co-morbidity (diabetes, heart disease) and postoperative mobilisation. Nevertheless, in a selected series of 343 day-case patients undergoing laparoscopic gastric banding, the unplanned overnight admission rate was 0.9%.[16] In a series of 50 patients randomised to day-case surgery or overnight stay, 76% of the day cases were successfully discharged the same day without re-admission.[17]

Breast cancer surgery

While benign breast disease is commonly performed on a day-case basis (duct excision, excision biopsy of cysts or fibroadenomas), there has been a reluctance in the UK to provide day-case breast surgery for breast cancer patients for both technical and psychological reasons.

Although selected patients undergoing simple mastectomy are able to return home the same day with suction drains *in situ*, the cost of the Breast Care Nurse in monitoring and removing the drains in the community remains prohibitive. Day-case wide local excision and axillary sampling without drainage has been reported,[18] but the introduction of sentinel lymph node biopsy, replacing axillary node dissection for patients with clinically negative nodes[19] has reduced the need for axillary drains and made the procedure an ideal day case.

The lingering belief that the breast cancer patient is best served by providing overnight or short-stay hospital support during their anxious and emotional peri-operative period often proves a barrier to day-case breast cancer surgery. However, it has been shown that patients undergoing surgery for breast cancer on an ambulatory basis, report faster recovery and better psychological adjustment.[20]

Endocrine surgery

1. **Parathyroid surgery** – Surgery for primary hyperparathyroidism has traditionally involved bilateral neck exploration performed as an in-patient. The newer concept of 'focused' parathyroidectomy has demonstrated 80% day-case rates for unifocal disease[21] when confirmed by sestamibi scanning and/or ultrasonography.[22] Through a small lateral incision, the adenomatous gland is removed and success is monitored by intra-operative parathyroid hormone measurement. Oral calcium supplements to prevent symptomatic hypocalcaemia are routinely given for 2 weeks postoperatively.

2. **Thyroid surgery** – The fear of postoperative haemorrhage leading to tracheal pressure has excluded traditional extensive necklace incisions for thyroid surgery from the day-surgery domain. However, the fact that most postoperative complications occur within 6 hours of operation[23] and the development of a minimal access approach to unilobular solitary nodules[24] creates the possibility of day-case thyroid surgery to selected patients. The incision (about 2.5 cm) is placed either transversely below the thyroid notch or more laterally. The use of the harmonic scalpel has facilitated faster surgery, minimal intra-operative haemorrhage and reduced postoperative blood loss into the drain, which can be removed easily where appropriate to allow same day discharge.[25]

3. **Laparoscopic adrenalectomy** – Laparoscopic adrenalectomy can be rapidly performed with operative times in selected patients under 1 hour[25] using the trans-abdominal lateral flank approach. This is appropriate for small tumours and patients with Conn's disease, not for patients with phaeochromocytoma. Although experience is at present limited, day-case surgery has been achieved but numbers remain small.[26]

Gallbladder surgery

While laparoscopic cholecystectomy is not a new day-case procedure, it is included here because it is a 'basket' procedure but the national average (England) day-case rate is only 6.4%.[27] Indeed, one-third of acute trusts perform no day-case laparoscopic cholecystectomies whatsoever. The reasons for poor uptake can be divided into clinical doubt, poorly designed clinical pathways and the organisation of surgical resources.

Clinical reasons for day-case reluctance relate to fears regarding reactionary haemorrhage, delayed haemorrhage and bile leak. Reactionary haemorrhage occurs within 4–6 hours of surgery and can be corrected within the working day if the surgery is performed before noon. Late haemorrhage usually occurs 3–4 days after operation and, even if the patient had been an in-patient, they would likely have gone home before the secondary haemorrhage occurred. It is rare for bile leaks to become apparent before 48 hours. Accessory duct injury is often insidious and diathermy injury of the biliary tree and stump leakage may take days to manifest. Again, if the patient had undergone in-patient surgery, the likelihood is that discharge to home would already have occurred.

Key point 6

- Reluctance to transfer in-patient procedures to the day unit is often the result of myth and misinformation rather than patient preference and peer review.

Attention to surgical detail enhances the prospect of successful day surgery. Carbon dioxide gas under the diaphragm creates shoulder tip pain and should be expelled from the abdomen before closure.[28] Blood in the peritoneal cavity is irritant and achieving a haemostatic liver bed is worthwhile. Even if a suction drain is inserted, it can often be removed within a few hours and the patient is still able to return home the same day.

The successful day-case laparoscopic cholecystectomy pathway relies on allowing the patient 4–8 hours' recovery before discharge.[29] Thus, procedures should be performed early in the operating list – later, and the case becomes an unplanned overnight admission. In the early days, unplanned admission rates were high; now, many units with a dedicated day-case laparoscopic chole-cystectomy programme demonstrated an acceptable rate between 5–10%.[30,31]

The procedure of laparoscopic cholecystectomy is now a standard training operation for the general surgical SpR. There is a danger of prolonged operating time during training and patients allocated to 23-hour surgery may be more appropriate. In many hospitals, laparoscopic cholecystectomy is performed by all general surgical consultants. However, a recent review recommends a minimum of 200 laparoscopic cholecystectomies per surgeon over 5 years to minimise conversion and complications and to improve outcomes. (This equates to a minimum of 40 cases per year.[32]) In many district general hospitals throughout the UK, work-load patterns preclude the development of a specialist service; there is no doubt that good outcomes, and good day-case outcomes especially, can only be achieved by a dedicated team at consultant level.

Laparoscopic incisional hernia repair

Open techniques for incisional/ventral hernia repair carry a high recurrence rate of 43%.[33] The use of prosthetic mesh by open technique reduces this incidence to 24%,[34] but open procedures often require extensive tissue dissection which increases complication rates. Laparoscopic incisional hernia repair confers significant advantages to the patient by avoiding an open abdominal wound[35] and offers the possibility of performing the procedure on a day-case basis. The mesh is placed against the underside of the abdominal wall with 3–5 cm circumferential overlap depending on the size of the defect. Using this sublay technique, the mesh is fixed in position with a variety of anchoring devices. Day-surgery rates for the procedure are disappointing at about 40%, perhaps due to the size of the defects repaired, but also anchoring devices inserted into the abdominal muscle appear to create a disproportionate degree of postoperative discomfort leading to an overnight stay. Nevertheless, successful series of day-case laparoscopic incisional hernia repairs have been reported and are acceptable to patients and cost-effective to the hospital.[35,36]

Laparoscopic splenectomy

The technique of laparoscopic splenectomy has been used for elective haematological and neoplastic conditions. Day-case rates of 83% of selected patients have been achieved.[37] The main barrier to day surgery is the exit incision for removal of the intact spleen, either by extending an existing trochar incision or creating a new portal in the left iliac fossa. Thus, there is a relative contra-indication to the removal of very large spleens, unless maceration is performed before excision.

Vascular surgery

1. **Varicose vein surgery** – Surgery for varicose veins has been part of the audit commission basket of vascular procedures since its inception in 1990. In many hospitals, varicose vein surgery has provided a successful, high-volume, day-surgery procedure to enable many trusts to achieve their day surgery 75% 'basket' target. Recent overt rationing of varicose vein surgery (restricting operations to those with severe symptoms, varicose eczema, or ulceration) has resulted in an older, less fit population with more severe venous disease. However, newer techniques for long and short saphenous vein obliteration (such as radiofrequency ablation, laser ablation and foam sclerotherapy) can be performed under local anaesthetic in a procedure room on a day-case basis without requiring full theatre facilities.[38–40]

2. **Thoracoscopic sympathectomy** – Although the indications for thoracoscopic sympathectomy are limited, the unilateral procedure lends itself to day surgery as it is commonly performed in less than half-an-hour, is minimally invasive and postoperative pain is minimal. The main indication is palmar and axillary hyperhidrosis although in some centres it is also performed for facial blushing and sweating, and occasionally for severe Raynaud's disease. A double-lumen endotracheal tube to allow individual lung ventilation is unnecessary as laryngeal mask anaesthesia is safe and the lung is deflated by inserting 600–800 ml of carbon dioxide by Veress needle into the thoracic cavity before trochar insertion. After transection of the sympathetic trunk over the neck of the second rib, the lung is re-inflated under direct vision. Many units no longer perform a

routine postoperative chest X-ray unless the oxygen saturation is reduced (< 92% on air), or if there is shortness of breath or chest pain.[41] The incidence of significant pneumothorax requiring chest drain and overnight admission is less than 1%.

THE FUTURE

The development of newer procedures for day surgery often begins with the short-stay pathway leading to 23-hour surgery before finally achieving day-surgery status. Many of the newer procedures for day surgery discussed in this article have followed this tried and tested route. Many other procedures are on the point of achieving day surgery breakthrough. In colorectal surgery, laparoscopic techniques have dramatically reduced the patient's stay for anterior resection or reversal of colostomy to 2–3 days. In vascular surgery, endovascular techniques for carotid stenting and abdominal aortic aneurysm stenting allow patients to be discharged within 48 hours. While safety considerations of the individual patient remain paramount, patient demand for shorter in-patient stay, the reduced incidence of MRSA in ambulatory patients, and the fiscal considerations of the Department of Health, will ensure that the drive towards day surgery will continue at an ever increasing pace.

Key points for clinical practice

- The NHS Plan indicated that the day surgery target should be 75% of the Audit Commission 'basket' of 25 procedures.

- Day-surgery rates remain lower than expected with the average for England (69.8%), Wales (60%) and Scotland (50%) all below 75%.

- The British Association of Day Surgery directory offers aspirational percentages for 160 short-stay procedures as out-patient procedures, day cases, 23-hour cases, short-stay cases (< 72 hours).

- Day surgery developments are the result of improvements in anaesthesia and analgesia as well as the surgery itself.

- Newer procedures for day surgery occur as a result of the introduction of new technologies and techniques, or revisiting traditional surgical procedures due to safer, extended-duration anaesthesia.

- Reluctance to transfer in-patient procedures to the day unit is often the result of myth and misinformation rather than patient preference and peer review.

References

1. Department of Health. *Day Surgery: Operational Guide.* London: Department of Health, 2002.
2. Audit Commission. *Day Surgery – Review of National Findings.* London: Audit Commission, 2001.

3. Dr. Foster's case notes. Trends in day surgery rates. *BMJ* 2005; 331: 803.

4. NHS Institute for Innovation and Improvement. *NHS better care, better value indicators.* London: NHS Institute for Innovation and Improvement, 2006.

5. Department of Health. *The NHS Plan: a plan for investment, a plan for reform.* London: Department of Health, 2000.

6. Scottish Executive. *The planned care improvement programme: Day surgery in Scotland.* Edinburgh: Scottish Executive, 2006.

7. Wales Audit Office. *Making better use of NHS day surgery in Wales.* Cardiff: Wales Audit Office, 2006.

8. British Association of Day Surgery. *BADS Directory of Procedures.* London: British Association of Day Surgery, 2006.

9. Anon. *Day Surgery*, revised edn. February 2005. <www.aagbio.org>.

10. Anon. *Acute Pain Management: Scientific Review.* Australian and New Zealand College of Anaesthetists and Faculty of Pain Medicine, 2005.

11. Claxton AR, McGuire G, Chung F, Cruise C. Evaluation of morphine versus fentanyl for post-operative analgesia after ambulatory surgical procedures. *Anesth Analg* 1997; **84**: 509–514.

12. Yogendran S, Asokumar B, Cheng DC, Chung F. A prospective randomised double-blinded study of the effect of intravenous fluid therapy on adverse outcomes on out-patient surgery. *Anesth Analg* 1995; **80**: 682–686.

13. Bandolier Website <www.jr2.ox.uk/bandolier/Extraforbando.combo.pdf>.

14. Skattum J, Edwin B, Trondsen E *et al.* Out-patient laparoscopic surgery: feasibility and consequences for education and health care costs. *Surg Endosc* 2004; **18**: 796–801

15. Bailey ME, Garrett WV, Nisar A, Boyle NH, Slater GH. Day-case laparoscopic Nissen fundoplication. *Br J Surg* 2003; **90**: 560–562.

16. Watkins BM, Montgomery KF, Ahroni JH *et al.* Adjustable gastric banding in an ambulatory center. *Obesity Surg* 2005; **15**: 1045–1049.

17. Wasowicz-Kemps DK, Bliemer B, Boom FA, de Zwaan NM, Van Ramshorst B. Laparoscopic gastric banding for morbid obesity: out-patient procedure versus overnight stay. *Surg Endosc* 2006; **20**: 1233–1237.

18. Athey N, Gilliam AD, Sinha P *et al.* Day-case breast cancer axillary surgery. *Ann R Coll Surg Engl* 2005; **87**: 96–98.

19. Ronka R, Smitten K, Sintonen H *et al.* The impact of sentinel node biopsy and axillary staging strategy on hospital costs. *Ann Oncol* 2004; **15**: 88–94.

20. Margolese RG, Lasry JC. Ambulatory surgery for breast cancer patients. *Ann Surg Oncol* 2000; **7**: 181–187.

21. Gurnelle EM. Thomas SK, McFarlane I *et al.* Focused parathyroid surgery with intra-operative parathyroid hormone measurement as a day case procedure. *Br J Surg* 2004; **91**: 78–82.

22. Carr ERM, Contractor K, Remedious D, Burke M. Can parathyroidectomy for primary hyperparathyroidism be carried out as a day case procedure? *J Laryngol Otol* 2006; **120**: 939–941.

23. Smith KG, Ridgeway LM, Mihaimeep F. A UK wide survey of post-operative thyroid surgical practice and life threatening complications. *Endocrine Abstracts* 2005; **10**: 94.

24. Palazzo FF, Sywak MS, Sidhu SB, Delbridge LW. Safety and feasibility of thyroid lobectomy via a lateral 2.5-cm incision with a cohort comparison of the first 50 cases: evolution of a surgical approach. *Arch Surg* 2005; **390**: 230–235.

25. Hopkins C, Mansuri S, Terry RM. How we do it: dispensing with drains in hemi-thyroidectomy – a feasibility study. *Clin Otolaryngol* 2006; **31**: 452–455.

26. Edwin B, Raeder I, Trondsen E, Kaaresen R, Buanes T. Out-patient laparoscopic adrenalectomy in patients with Conn's syndrome. *Surg Endosc* 2001; **15**: 589–591.

27. NHS Institute for Innovation and Improvement. *Focus on Cholecystectomy.* London: Department of Health, 2006.

28. Jackson SA, Lawrence AS, Hill JC. Does post-laparoscopy pain relate to residual carbon dioxide? *Anaesthesia* 1996; 51: 485–487.

29. McWhinnie D, Ellams J, Cahill J, Smith I. *Day case laparoscopic cholecystectomy.* London: British Association of Day Surgery, 2004.

30. Huang A, Stinchcombe C, Davis M, Phillips D, McWhinnie DL. Prospective five year audit for day case laparoscopic cholecystectomy. *J One Day Surg* 2000; **9**: 15–17.

31. Leeder PC, Matthews T, Krzeminska K, Dehn TC. Routine day case laparoscopic cholecystectomy. *Br J Surg* 2004; **91**: 312–316.
32. Hobbs MS, Mai Q, Knuiman MW, Fletcher DR, Ridout CS. Surgeon experience and trends in intra-operative complications in laparoscopic cholecystectomy. *Br J Surg* 2006; **93**: 844–853.
33. Luijendijk RW, Hop WL, Van Den Tol MP *et al*. A comparison of suture repair with mesh repair for incisional hernia. *N Engl J Med* 2000; **342**: 392–398.
34. Pollak R, Nyhos LM. Incisional hernias. In:Schwarz SI, Ellis H. (eds) *Maingot's Abdominal Operations*, 8th edn, vol 1. Norwack: Appleton-Century-Crofts, 1985; 335–350.
35. Engledow AH, Sengupta N, Akhras F, Tutton M, Warren SJ. Day case laparoscopic incisional hernia repair is feasible, acceptable and cost effective. *Surg Endosc* 2007; **21**: 84–86.
36. Heniford BT, Park A, Ramshaw BJ, Voeller G. Laparoscopic ventral and incisional hernia repair in 407 patients. *J Am Coll Surg* 2000; **190**: 645–650.
37. Edwin B, Skattum J, Raeder J, Trundsen E, Baunes T. Out-patient laparoscopic splenectomy: patient safety and satisfaction. *Surg Endosc* 2004; **18**: 1331–1334.
38. Lurie F, Eklof B, Kabnik LS *et al*. Prospective randomised study of endovenous radiofrequency obliteration versus ligation and stripping in a selected patient population. *J Vasc Surg* 2003; **38**: 207–214.
39. Min RJ, Zimmer SE. Endovenous laser treatment of saphenous vein reflux. *J Vasc Interview Radiol* 2004; **15**: 203.
40. Bradbury A. Foam sclerotherapy for the treatment of varicose veins. In: Heshiren JM, Taylor P, Thompson M. (eds) *Advancing the boundaries of vascular surgical practice*, vol. 29. Sheffield: Aesculap Academia, 2005; 1–9.
41. Cameron A. How I do endoscopic sympathectomy. In: Cheshire N, Jenkins M. Taylor P, Thompson M. (eds) *Advancing the boundaries of vascular surgical practice*, vol. 25. Sheffield: Aesculap Academia, 2005; 1–7.

Narasimhaiah Srinivasaiah Philip J. Drew

5

Quality of life issues in breast surgery

Evaluation of quality of life (QoL) is an important measured outcome in the field of breast surgery. Health-related quality of life (HRQoL) is also an important end-point in cancer treatment. However, a relatively small proportion of professionals truly understand the concepts and uses of QoL assessments.

HEALTH

In 1948, the World Health Organization (WHO), in its Constitution, defined health as: 'A state of complete physical, mental, and social well-being and not merely the absence of disease or infirmity'. Health is multidimensional (physical, mental, social, and role). It is important to quantify these health indicators/measures. In addition to the traditional indicators of healthcare outcome namely mortality, morbidity and cost, personal assessments of functional status and well-being, customers' reports, ratings of care, services, and health plans are all driving towards a patient-based assessment. Ware et al.[1] defined QoL as:

> *Quality of life is a state of mind ... how good it is to you, and only you can decide that. If I want to know your quality of life, I have to ask you. I can't know it by observing you; I have to ask you. And that's the way we gather quality of life data. The health-related quality of life is that part of your quality of life that is more affected by disease and health care treatment.*

Narasimhaiah Srinivasaiah MRCS(Eng.) MRCS(Ed.) MRCPS(Glasg.) MRCSI MD (DNB – India)
Research Fellow, Academic Surgical Unit, University of Hull, Castle Hill Hospital, Cottingham, Hull HU16 4AY, UK

Philip J. Drew BSc MD MS FRCS(Eng.) FRCS(Ed.) FRCPS(Glasg.) (for correspondence)
Professor, Hull York Medical School, Castle Hill Hospital, Cottingham, Hull HU16 4AY, UK
E-mail: p.j.drew@hull.ac.uk

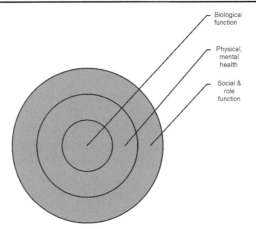

Biological
function

Physical,
mental
health

Social &
role
function

Fig. 1 Health concepts (after Ware et al.[1]).

Disruption in any of these dimensions of health can compromise functioning and well-being in other areas. Ill health can come from anywhere, but all of these states must be in balance in order to have perfect health.

QoL AND HRQoL

It is important to understand the distinction between QoL and HRQoL. QoL is a global concept with many themes, including overall satisfaction with life as well as the specific domains of life including family, community, work, and health. HRQoL takes into account the values of the individual, narrowing the focus to health concepts, such as functioning, that are affected by disease and treatment.[2]

HEALTH SURVEYS

Outcomes research examines the end results of medical interventions, taking into account patients' experiences, preferences, and values. The purpose of assessing outcomes is to provide evidence on which to base clinical decisions. Health surveys are tools used for evaluating various concepts of health and to provide a patient-based assessment of health. They are broadly categorised into generic and specific health measures.

GENERIC HEALTH MEASURES

Generic health measures assess health concepts that represent basic human values and are relevant to everyone's health status and well-being, regardless

Table 1 Generic health measures

- European Quality of Life Index (EuroQoL)
- MOS Short Forms (SF-36 and SF-12)
- Nottingham Health Profile (NHP)
- Quality of Well-Being Scale (QWB)
- Sickness Impact Profile (SIP)
- Health Utilities Index (HUI)
- Quality-of-Life Index
- Subjective quality of life profile (SQLP)
- General health questionnaire (GHQ12)

of age, disease, or treatment group (Table 1).[3] For the purpose of illustration, let us look at one of them.

Medical Outcome Study (MOS) Short Forms (SF-36 and SF-12)

The SF-36 was designed to serve as a core general health measure, the 36-item survey, which requires 6–9 minutes on average to complete. Survey items capture eight health concepts (physical functioning, role-physical, bodily pain, general health, vitality, social functioning, role-emotional, and mental health).

Table 2 Specific health measures

Breast
Breast Evaluation Questionnaire
Breast Chest Ratings Scale (BCRS)
Derriford Scale (DAS59)
Multidimensional Body-States Relations Questionnaire (MBSRQ)

Cancer
Cancer Functional Living Index for Cancer
European Organization for Research and Treatment of Cancer (EORTC)
Functional Assessment of Cancer Therapy for Breast Cancer (FACT-B)
Mental adjustment to cancer (MAC) scale
Cancer Rehabilitation Evaluation System (CARES-SF)
Functional living index-cancer (FLIC)

Psychosocial
Psychosocial Adjustment to Illness Scale
Courtauld Emotional Control (CEC) scale
Folkman and Lazarus Ways of Coping Questionnaire
Modified Folkman and Lazarus Ways of Coping Questionnaire
Profile of Mood States
LOT-R – Measure of optimism
Hospital Anxiety and Depression Score

Pain
Pain Disability Questionnaire
McGill Pain Questionnaire
MOS Pain Measures

Illness/survivorship
Adaptation to survivorship
Mischel Uncertainty in Illness Scale

Scale construction studies support several scoring options, including a profile of health states across the eight concepts, summary measures of physical and of mental health outcomes, and a single utility index of health. Published scoring algorithms include data quality checks. Results of extensive validity studies have been published, and norm based scoring further improves the interpretation of scores.

SPECIFIC HEALTH MEASURES

Specific measures focus on the particulars of a specific disease or diagnostic group (*e.g.* cancer), condition (*e.g.* congestive heart failure), or treatment (*e.g.* hip replacement), and are designed to capture areas of health specifically affected by that disease or treatment.[4] Some of the specific health measures used are shown in Table 2 above.

Key point 2

- QoL and HRQoL are two different entities. Health surveys are important tools for evaluating various concepts of health and provide patient-based assessment of health. They are broadly categorised into generic and specific health measures.

The magnitude of aesthetic and oncoplastic surgical work in relation to breast is on the rise. A brief discussion of the QoL issues is outlined below.

ONCOPLASTIC SURGERY AND QoL ISSUES

Following surgery, younger women experience a lower QoL due to the effects of medical treatment.[5] The effects of surgery and removal of the breast result in more negative feelings regarding body image.[5] Systemic treatment make many younger women experience the sudden onset of menopause and relationship issues contributing to a high level of sexual concern. Psychosocially, it affects both females and their partners. Emotional support from the partner is important in women's adjustment. There is encouraging evidence that couple-based psychosocial interventions might be of particular assistance to both partners.[5]

In a Far-East study looking at early effect of surgery on QoL in women with operable breast cancer, patients were interviewed prior to and after the surgery using FACT-B. There was no significant change in overall QoL immediately after the surgery, probably reflecting strong family and social support for these women. Similar results have been reported by studies from other countries.[6]

Young women after breast-conserving surgery and radiation therapy experience changes in QoL, psychosocial adjustment, and adaptation to survivorship issues during radiation therapy. Changes may not reflect what is observed in clinical practice. As such, there is a need to understand and support young women during radiation therapy.[7]

Schultz *et al.*[8] studied the QoL issues in long-term survivors of breast cancer. They concluded that breast cancer and menopause are independent issues and should not be confused with the QoL/psychosocial issues of the cancer survivor. Understanding these issues is important to provide holistic nursing care.

Casso et al.[9] examined the correlates of QoL of a well-defined group of 5–10-year breast cancer survivors diagnosed between the ages of 40 and 49 years using questionnaires. CARES-SF and SF-36 were some of the measures used. Breast-related symptoms, use of adjuvant therapy, lower income, and type of breast surgery were significantly associated with lower QoL 5–10 years post-diagnosis. The authors emphasised that younger, long-term survivors have a high QoL across several standardised measures. The long-term consequences of adjuvant therapy and management of long-term breast-related symptoms are two areas that may be important for clinicians and women with breast cancer in understanding and optimising long-term QoL.

A survey done among members of the British Association of Surgical Oncology to frame the attitude and perception of breast surgeons in the UK demonstrated age as not a criterion in identifying a patient as elderly in 44%.[10] The surgeons felt that the decision-making process was based on multiple factors to tailor the most appropriate treatment aiming to improving QoL (42%) and quality adjusted survival (40%). No routine geriatric assessment was used (82%). The survey confirmed lack of knowledge in the management of elderly patients affected by breast cancer.

Key point 3

- Breast surgery results in more negative feelings regarding body image. Younger women experience a lower QoL due to the effects of medical treatment. Psychosocially, breast cancer affects both females and their partners. Support from the partner is important in women's adjustment. There is a lack of knowledge in the management of elderly patients affected by breast cancer.

RECONSTRUCTIVE SURGERY AND QoL

Reconstructive surgery plays an important role in physical and emotional outcome among breast cancer survivors. The psychosocial impact of primary surgery occurs largely in areas of body image and feelings of attractiveness, with women receiving lumpectomy experiencing the most positive outcome.[11] The type of primary surgery has no significance on emotional, social, or role function.[11] Beyond the first year after diagnosis, a woman's quality of life is more likely influenced by her age or exposure to adjuvant therapy than by her breast surgery.[11] In the case of mastectomy, reconstruction will restore lost femininity, sexuality, and normality in most cases, not because of the procedure but because of elimination of prostheses.[12]

Older patients do well when it comes to mental health scores compared to younger women post reconstruction. Girotto et al.[13] studied breast reconstruction after mastectomy in women older than 65 years of age and its impact on QoL. SF-36 outcome measure was used. Older patients scored lower (worse outcomes) in the areas related to physical function and maintained superior scores (better outcomes) over the younger patients in the subscales influenced by mental health.

In breast cancer, apart from improving disease-free survival, QoL, body image and cosmetic outcome are important issues. Cocquyt et al.[14] evaluated HRQoL and body image in patients treated with pre-operative chemotherapy followed by breast conserving surgery, or skin-sparing mastectomy and perforator-flap breast reconstruction. Participants were evaluated by SF-36 and a study-specific questionnaire. The authors showed that breast conserving treatment or mastectomy with reconstruction may yield comparable results of QoL, but cosmetic outcome was better after skin-sparing mastectomy and perforator-flap reconstruction. Patients must be offered both options, and clinicians should stress that both are equally effective.

QoL, patients' satisfaction, and aesthetic outcome after pedicled or free TRAM flap breast surgery were studied to evaluate the aesthetic result of the breast reconstruction both objectively and subjectively.[15] No statistically significant difference between pedicle and free TRAM flap was seen in surgical groups regarding patient satisfaction with the reconstruction. In the patients' self-assessment of the cosmetic outcome, the degree of symmetry was assessed higher in the free TRAM flap group. SF-36 revealed no difference between the pedicled and free flap groups. A strong correlation between patient and panel evaluation of the cosmetic outcome was seen.

The psychosocial impact of breast surgery has been extensively studied in the West. There is a relative paucity of comparable data in oriental women who are increasingly affected by cancer of the breast. Fung et al.[16] studied the effects that different types of breast surgery have on the QoL of Chinese women. Aspects of QoL measured included general psychological well-being, body image, sexual and social function. The results showed that breast-conserving treatment had significantly improved body image scores compared to mastectomy. The three groups – breast-conserving treatment, mastectomy, and mastectomy with immediate breast reconstruction – did not differ significantly in the other aspects of quality of life measured.

Nissen et al.[17] looked at women's expectations following mastectomy reconstruction and factors affecting their QoL. Qualitative focus groups revealed women wished they had been better informed about some issues. Ratings of satisfaction generally were high. There were concerns about cosmetic outcome and persistent anxiety about recurrence. Women appreciated information to prepare them for reconstruction and recovery.

QoL after breast carcinoma surgery when compared between breast conservation surgery, mastectomy alone, and mastectomy with reconstruction was shown to be equal for the treatment of early stage breast carcinoma using the Mischel Uncertainty in Illness Scale, Profile of Mood States, and FACT for Breast Cancer.[18] In conclusion, aspects of QoL other than body image were not better in women who underwent breast conservation surgery or mastectomy with reconstruction than in women who had mastectomy alone. Mastectomy with reconstruction was associated with greater mood disturbance and poorer well-being.[18]

Harcourt et al.[19] examined the research literature relating to the psychological aspects of breast reconstruction. Particular attention was given to the role of specialist breast care nurses and psychological benefits. There is a lack of studies examining breast reconstruction in terms of relevant psychological constructs, especially in relation to coping and decision-making. They concluded that existing research into the psychological aspects of breast reconstruction is limited and not sufficiently conclusive to inform changes to policy and the provision of care.

Key point 4

- Reconstructive surgery plays an important role in physical and emotional outcomes among breast cancer survivors. QoL other than body image is no better in women who undergo breast conservation surgery or mastectomy with reconstruction than in women who have mastectomy alone.

COMPLICATIONS AND QoL

Lymphoedema and post-mastectomy pain are complications that can have an impact on the QoL. Patients with lymphoedema may experience pain and body image issues. Complete decongestive therapy is effective in treating lymphoedema. The FACT- (QoL) measure and a visual analogue scale for pain showed successful reduction in girth, volume, and pain with increased QoL. QoL and pain are improved by treatment and continue to improve after the treatment has ended.[20]

Pain after quadrantectomy and radiotherapy for early-stage breast cancer affecting the QoL was studied using self-completed questionnaires.[21] The outcome measures used were McGill Pain Questionnaire and a QoL questionnaire. The authors supported the hypothesis that pain is a frequent sequelae of breast conservation surgery and radiotherapy, and that such symptoms can cause postoperative psychosocial distress, thus limiting patient adaptation and reducing the beneficial effect of breast conservation surgery on body image.

Macdonald et al.[22] looked at long-term follow-up of breast cancer survivors with post-mastectomy pain at 7–12 years' postoperatively. Chronic pain and QoL were assessed using the McGill Pain Questionnaire (MPQ) and SF-36. QoL scores were significantly lower in women with persistent post-mastectomy pain compared to those women whose pain had resolved.

Key point 5

- Lymphoedema and post-mastectomy pain have an impact on the QoL. Complete decongestive therapy is effective in treating lymphoedema.

PSYCHOLOGICAL FACTORS

In breast cancer, the psychological response to breast cancer, such as a fighting spirit or an attitude of helplessness and hopelessness toward the disease, has been suggested as a prognostic factor.

Watson *et al.*,[23] in a population-based study investigated the effect of psychological response on disease outcome in a large cohort of women with early-stage breast cancer. Psychological response was measured by the mental adjustment to cancer (MAC) scale, the Courtauld emotional control (CEC) scale, and the hospital anxiety and depression (HAD) scale. The authors found that for 5-year, event-free survival, a high helplessness/hopelessness score has a moderate detrimental effect. There were no significant results found for the category of 'fighting spirit'. A high score for depression is linked to a significantly reduced chance of survival.

Watson *et al.*[24] assessed the psychological responses of helplessness/hopelessness, fighting spirit and depression in early-stage breast cancer patients between 1 and 3 months' post-diagnosis. In order to ascertain the effect on cancer prognosis, patients were followed up for 10 years. There was a continuing effect of helplessness/hopelessness on disease-free survival, but not of depression. Longer follow-up also indicated that a high fighting spirit conferred no survival advantage. The results showed that, in patients who were disease-free at 5 years, baseline helpless/hopeless response still exerted a significant effect on disease-free survival beyond 5 years (and up to 10 years). The effect is, therefore, maintained for up to 10 years.

Reynolds *et al.*[25] evaluated the association between coping strategies and breast cancer survival among Black and White women. An emotion-focused coping strategy was associated with survival. Expression of emotion was associated with better survival suggesting that the opportunity for emotional expression may improve survival among patients with invasive breast cancer.

In a qualitative study by Cunningham and Watson,[26] common themes emerged: (i) 'authenticity', or a clear understanding of what was important in one's life; (ii) the perceived freedom to shape life around what was valued; and (iii) 'acceptance', a perceived change in mental state to enhanced self-esteem, greater tolerance for and emotional closeness to others, and an affective experience described as more peaceful and joyous. The authors also looked into the concept of remarkable survivors. They found a mirrored symmetry between the psychological patterns possibly promoting disease and the changed adaptations that may lead to longer survival in some cases. The authors suggested that the progression of cancer, or other chronic disease, is favoured by a distorted psychological adaptation and that healing may be assisted by a reversal of that adaptation in the case of cancer, toward greater authenticity of thought and action.[26]

Petticrew,[27] in a systematic review, analysed the influence of psychological coping on survival and recurrence in people with cancer and summarised the evidence that psychological coping styles (including fighting spirit, helplessness, hopelessness, denial, and avoidance) affect survival and recurrence in patients with cancer. He concluded that there is little consistent evidence that psychological coping styles play an important part in survival or recurrence. People with cancer should not feel pressured into adopting particular coping styles to improve survival or reduce the risk of recurrence. Although the relation is biologically plausible, there is, at present, little scientific basis for the popular lay and clinical belief that psychological coping styles have an important influence on overall or event-free survival in patients with cancer.

Key point 6

- Psychological responses such as a fighting spirit, helplessness and hopelessness have been suggested as a prognostic factor with an influence on survival. Little consistent evidence that psychological coping styles play an important part in survival from or recurrence of cancer has been shown by systematic reviews.

SERVICE PROVISIONS AND QoL

DAY-CASE SURGERY AND ROLE OF NURSES

Margolese *et al.*[28] compared in-patient to same-day discharge surgery for breast cancer on unselected patients. Out-patients and hospitalised patients reported similar levels of pain, fear, anxiety, health assessment, and QoL. Ambulatory patients manifested a significantly better emotional adjustment and fewer psychological distress symptoms. Same-day discharge patients are not at a disadvantage compared to hospitalised patients, *i.e.* they report faster recovery and better psychological adjustment. Out-patient surgery may thus foster patient emotional well-being better than routine hospitalisation.

Education for women being fitted for breast prostheses is best done by nurses who are instrumental in educating women about issues related to breast surgery and in helping to promote psychosocial adjustment. Prostheses and bras that fit properly can be very important in the recovery process and ultimately improve QoL.[29]

Key point 7

- Day-case patients report faster recovery and better psychological adjustment. Breast care nurses help in promotion of psycho-social adjustment and aid in improvement of QoL.

PHYSICAL EXERCISE AND QoL

Aerobics and resistance training exercises can improve the QoL for women recovering from breast cancer treatment. Long-term fatigue with subsequent decrease in QoL is also a serious problem for cancer survivors. Up to 30% may experience this symptom for years after termination of treatment.[30]

Key point 8

- Aerobics and resistance training exercises can improve the QoL for women recovering from breast cancer treatment.

COMPLEMENTARY AND ALTERNATIVE THERAPIES AND QoL

Yoga is a Sanskrit word meaning union; it refers to the union of the body, mind and spirit. Studies have shown that breast cancer patients who do yoga tend to enjoy better health, less fatigue and experience less daytime sleepiness. Short yoga programmes (including meditation, relaxation, breathing exercises, stretching, imagery and physical movements) have been shown to be useful at reducing the side-effects that come with breast cancer treatment.

Shannahoff-Khalsa[31] showed that the Kundalini yoga meditation technique for psycho-oncology is a potential therapy for patients with anxiety and depression. A pilot study[32] of yoga for breast cancer survivors showed physical and psychological benefits of lessening the impact of detrimental cancer-related symptoms and treatment side-effects (*e.g.* fatigue, nausea), and improving overall well-being and QoL.

Carlson *et al.*[33] investigated the relationships between mindfulness-based stress reduction (MBSR) in relation to QoL, mood, symptoms of stress, and immune parameters in breast and prostate cancer out-patients. The participants were enrolled into an 8-week MBSR programme that incorporated relaxation, meditation, gentle yoga, and daily home practice. Demographic and health behaviour variables, quality of life (EORTC QLQ C-30), mood (POMS), stress (SOSI), and counts of NK, NKT, B, T total, T helper, and T cytotoxic cells, as well as NK and T cell production of TNF, IFN-γ, IL-4, and IL-10 were assessed pre- and post-intervention. The authors concluded that MBSR participation was associated with enhanced QoL and decreased stress symptoms in breast and prostate cancer patients. This study is also the first to show changes in cancer-related cytokine production associated with programme participation.

In another study, Carlson *et al.*[34] concluded that MBSR programme enrolment was associated with enhanced QoL and decreased stress symptoms in breast and prostate cancer patients, and resulted in possibly beneficial changes in hypothalamic-pituitary-adrenal (HPA) axis functioning.

Key point 9

- Yoga proved to have physical and psychological benefits of lessening the impact of detrimental cancer-related symptoms and treatment side-effects. Mindfulness-based stress reduction participation was associated with enhanced QoL and decreased stress symptoms.

HEALTH OUTCOME MEASURES SPECIFIC TO BREAST CANCER

There are a few generic and specific health outcome measures used in breast surgery. Reliable and valid assessment instruments in cosmetic surgery are a vital factor in assessing patient satisfaction with physical appearance. Appearance and satisfaction assessments are needed to evaluate QoL adequately. The Breast Evaluation Questionnaire was designed to assess satisfaction with breast attributes. It is a 55-item questionnaire with subscales including comfort not fully dressed, comfort fully dressed, and satisfaction with breast attributes. The assessment is easy to administer and interpret and is recommended for assessing outcomes among breast augmentation patients, breast reconstruction patients, mastectomy patients, lumpectomy/breast-sparing surgery patients, breast reduction patients, and patients who have sustained trauma or injury to their breasts.[35]

Ching *et al.*,[36] in their literature review on measuring outcomes in aesthetic surgery, identified body-image and QoL measures to be of the greatest value in determining cosmetic surgery outcomes. These conclusions were based on a critical evaluation of the feasibility, validity, reliability, and sensitivity to change of these measures. The Multidimensional Body-States Relations Questionnaire (MBSRQ), a psychological assessment of body image, was selected as a potential candidate for further study. Breast Chest Ratings Scale (BCRS) was said to be useful in the assessment of breast surgery. The Derriford Scale (DAS59), an instrument that assesses appearance-related quality of life, was also selected. In addition, the authors recommend the use of a generic, utility-based quality-of-life instrument, such as the Health Utilities Index (HUI) EuroQol (EQ-5D).

Key point 10

- Reliable and valid assessment instruments in breast surgery are a vital factor in assessing patient satisfaction with physical appearance. The Breast Evaluation Questionnaire was designed to assess satisfaction with breast attributes.

Key points for clinical practice

- Health is multidimensional (physical, mental, and social role). Lack of an equilibrium among these entities leads to ill health. It is important to quantify these health indicators or measures.

- QoL and HRQoL are two different entities. Health surveys are important tools for evaluating various concepts of health and provide patient-based assessment of health. They are broadly categorised into generic and specific health measures.

- Breast surgery results in more negative feelings regarding body image. Younger women experience a lower QoL due to the effects of medical treatment. Psychosocially, breast cancer affects both females and their partners. Support from the partner is important in women's adjustment. Social and family support has a positive effect on QoL in the early postoperative period. There is a lack of knowledge in the management of elderly patients affected by breast cancer.

- Reconstructive surgery plays an important role in physical and emotional outcomes among breast cancer survivors. QoL other than body image is not better in women who undergo breast-conserving surgery or mastectomy with reconstruction than in women who have mastectomy alone. *(continued)*

Key points for clinical practice *(continued)*

- Lymphoedema and post-mastectomy pain have an impact on the QoL. Complete decongestive therapy is effective in treating lymphoedema.

- Psychological responses such as a fighting spirit, helplessness and hopelessness have been suggested as a prognostic factor with an influence on survival. Little consistent evidence that psychological coping styles play an important part in survival from or recurrence of cancer has been shown by systematic reviews.

- Day-case patients report faster recovery and better psychological adjustment. Breast care nurses help in promotion of psychosocial adjustment and aid in improvement of QoL.

- Aerobics and resistance training exercises can improve the QoL for women recovering from breast cancer treatment.

- Yoga proved to have physical and psychological benefits of lessening the impact of detrimental cancer-related symptoms and treatment side-effects. Mindfulness-based stress reduction participation was associated with enhanced QoL and decreased stress symptoms.

- Reliable and valid assessment instruments in breast surgery are a vital factor in assessing patient satisfaction with physical appearance. The Breast Evaluation Questionnaire was designed to assess satisfaction with breast attributes..

References

1. Ware Jr JE. on health status and quality of life assessment and the next generation of outcomes measurement. Interview by Marcia Stevic and Katie Berry. *J Health Qual* 1999; **21**: 12–17.
2. Patrick DPE. *Health Status and Health Policy: Quality of Life in Health Care Evaluation and Resource Allocation.* New York: Oxford University Press, 1993; 478.
3. Stewart AL. *Measuring Functioning and Well Being: The Medical Outcomes Study Approach.* Durham, NC: Duke University Press, 1992.
4. Bungay KM. *Measuring and Monitoring Health-Related Quality of Life: Current Concepts.* Kalamazoo, MI: Upjohn, 1993.
5. Baucom DH, Porter LS, Kirby JS *et al.* Psychosocial issues confronting young women with breast cancer. *Breast Dis* 2005; **23**: 103–113.
6. Pandey M, Thomas BC, Ramdas K, Ratheesan K. Early effect of surgery on quality of life in women with operable breast cancer. *Jpn J Clin Oncol* 2006; **36**: 468–472.
7. Dow KH, Lafferty P. Quality of life, survivorship, and psychosocial adjustment of young women with breast cancer after breast-conserving surgery and radiation therapy. *Oncol Nurs Forum* 2000; **27**: 1555–1564.
8. Schultz PN, Klein MJ, Beck ML *et al.* Breast cancer: relationship between menopausal symptoms, physiologic health effects of cancer treatment and physical constraints on quality of life in long-term survivors. *J Clin Nurs* 2005; **14**: 204–211.
9. Casso D, Buist DS, Taplin S. Quality of life of 5–10 year breast cancer survivors diagnosed between age 40 and 49. *Health Qual Life Outcomes* 2004; **2**: 25.
10. Audisio RA, Osman N, Audisio MM, Montalto F. How do we manage breast cancer in

the elderly patients? A survey among members of the British Association of Surgical Oncologists (BASO). *Crit Rev Oncol Hematol* 2004; **52**: 135–141.

11. Rowland JH, Desmond KA, Meyerowitz BE *et al*. Role of breast reconstructive surgery in physical and emotional outcomes among breast cancer survivors. *J Natl Cancer Inst* 2000; **92**: 1422–1429.

12. Crompvoets S. Comfort, control, or conformity: women who choose breast reconstruction following mastectomy. *Health Care Women Int* 2006; **27**: 75–93.

13. Girotto JA, Schreiber J, Nahabedian MY. Breast reconstruction in the elderly: preserving excellent quality of life. *Ann Plast Surg* 2003; **50**: 572–578.

14. Cocquyt VF, Blondeel PN, Depypere HT *et al*. Better cosmetic results and comparable quality of life after skin-sparing mastectomy and immediate autologous breast reconstruction compared to breast conservative treatment. *Br J Plast Surg* 2003; **56**: 462–470.

15. Edsander-Nord A, Brandberg Y, Wickman M. Quality of life, patients' satisfaction, and aesthetic outcome after pedicled or free TRAM flap breast surgery. *Plast Reconstr Surg* 2001; **107**: 1142–1154.

16. Fung KW, Lau Y, Fielding R *et al*. The impact of mastectomy, breast-conserving treatment and immediate breast reconstruction on the quality of life of Chinese women. *Aust NZ J Surg* 2001; **71**: 202–206.

17. Nissen MJ, Swenson KK, Kind EA. Quality of life after postmastectomy breast reconstruction. *Oncol Nurs Forum* 2002; **29**: 547–553.

18. Nissen MJ, Swenson KK, Ritz LJ *et al*. Quality of life after breast carcinoma surgery: a comparison of three surgical procedures. *Cancer* 2001; **91**: 1238–1246.

19. Harcourt D, Rumsey N. Psychological aspects of breast reconstruction: a review of the literature. *J Adv Nurs* 2001; **35**: 477–487.

20. Mondry TE, Riffenburgh RH, Johnstone PA. Prospective trial of complete decongestive therapy for upper extremity lymphedema after breast cancer therapy. *Cancer J* 2004; **10**: 42–49.

21. Amichetti M, Caffo O. Pain after quadrantectomy and radiotherapy for early-stage breast cancer: incidence, characteristics and influence on quality of life. Results from a retrospective study. *Oncology* 2003; **65**: 23–28.

22. Macdonald L, Bruce J, Scott NW *et al*. Long-term follow-up of breast cancer survivors with post-mastectomy pain syndrome. *Br J Cancer* 2005; **92**: 225–230.

23. Watson M, Haviland JS, Greer S *et al*. Influence of psychological response on survival in breast cancer: a population-based cohort study. *Lancet* 1999; **354**: 1331–1336.

24. Watson M, Homewood J, Haviland J, Bliss JM. Influence of psychological response on breast cancer survival: 10-year follow-up of a population-based cohort. *Eur J Cancer* 2005; **41**: 1710–1714.

25. Reynolds P, Hurley S, Torres M *et al*. Use of coping strategies and breast cancer survival: results from the Black/White Cancer Survival Study. *Am J Epidemiol* 2000; **152**: 940–949.

26. Cunningham AJ, Watson K. How psychological therapy may prolong survival in cancer patients: new evidence and a simple theory. *Integr Cancer Ther* 2004; **3**: 214–229.

27. Petticrew M, Bell R, Hunter D. Influence of psychological coping on survival and recurrence in people with cancer: systematic review. *BMJ* 2002; **325**: 1066.

28. Margolese RG, Lasry JC. Ambulatory surgery for breast cancer patients. *Ann Surg Oncol* 2000; **7**: 181–187.

29. Mahon SM, Casey M. Patient education for women being fitted for breast prostheses. *Clin J Oncol Nurs* 2003; **7**: 194–199.

30. Herrero FBJ, Balmer J, San Juan AF, Foster C *et al*. Is cardiorespiratory fitness related to quality of life in survivors of breast cancer? *J Strength Cond Res* 2006; **20**(3):535–540.

31. Shannahoff-Khalsa DS. Patient perspectives: Kundalini yoga meditation techniques for psycho-oncology and as potential therapies for cancer. *Integr Cancer Ther* 2005; **4**: 87–100.

32. Culos-Reed NS, Carlson LE, Daroux LM, Hately-Aldous S. A pilot study of yoga for breast cancer survivors: physical and psychological benefits. *Psychooncology* 2006; **15**: 891–897.

33. Carlson LE, Speca M, Patel KD, Goodey E. Mindfulness-based stress reduction in relation to quality of life, mood, symptoms of stress, and immune parameters in breast and prostate cancer outpatients. *Psychosom Med* 2003; **65**: 571–581.

34. Carlson LE, Speca M, Patel KD, Goodey E. Mindfulness-based stress reduction in relation to quality of life, mood, symptoms of stress and levels of cortisol, dehydroepiandrosterone sulfate (DHEAS) and melatonin in breast and prostate cancer outpatients. *Psychoneuroendocrinology* 2004; **29**: 448–474.
35. Anderson RC, Cunningham B, Tafesse E, Lenderking WR. Validation of the breast evaluation questionnaire for use with breast surgery patients. *Plast Reconstr Surg* 2006; **118**: 597–602.
36. Ching S, Thoma A, McCabe RE, Antony MM. Measuring outcomes in aesthetic surgery: a comprehensive review of the literature. *Plast Reconstr Surg* 2003; **111**: 469-481.

Author query

30. Please check reference?

José A. Cid Fernández John F.R. Robertson
D. Mark Sibbering

6

The management of high-risk familial breast cancer

Breast cancer is the commonest cancer in the UK, with over 40,000 new cases diagnosed and about 13,000 deaths per annum.[1] The exact causes of breast cancer remain unclear. One of the strongest risk factors for the development of breast cancer is the presence of a family history of the disease, although only 10–20% of affected women report such a history.[2] Familial clustering may result from genetic predisposition, but it may also be a consequence of shared physical environment and lifestyle or even from the operation of chance. In most populations, specific cancer susceptibility genes appear directly responsible for about 5% of all breast cancers.[3]

It is not yet known how many breast cancer predisposition genes there may be. Two autosomal dominant breast cancer genes, *BRCA1* and *BRCA2*, have been identified and these account for a considerable proportion of all hereditary breast cancer. The genes are associated with a high risk of developing breast, ovarian, and other cancers. Identification of high-risk women with a strong family history of the disease and, whenever possible, identification of gene mutation carriers is thus important as it allows for individualised risk reduction interventions.

THE *BRCA1* AND *BRCA2* GENES

In the last decade, the *BRCA1* and *BRCA2* genes were identified on the long arms of chromosomes 17 and 13, respectively. *BRCA1* accounts for the majority

José A. Cid Fernández DM FRCS
Specialist Registrar, Professorial Unit of Surgery, Nottingham City Hospital, Hucknall Road, Nottingham NG5 1PB, UK

John F.R. Robertson MD FRCS
Professor of Surgery, University of Nottingham, Nottingham City Hospital, Hucknall Road, Nottingham NG5 1PB, UK

D. Mark Sibbering FRCS (for correspondence)
Consultant Breast Surgeon, Department of Breast Surgery, Derby City General Hospital, Uttoxeter Road, Derby DE22 3NE, UK
E-mail: mark.sibbering@derbyhospitals.nhs.uk

of families with breast and ovarian cancer; in families with male breast cancer, BRCA2 mutations are more common.[4,5] The highest population prevalence rates of BRCA mutation carrier frequencies are found in Ashkenazi Jews, with 2.5% (1 in 40) of the population carrying one of three recurrent mutations in these genes, accounting for 12% of all breast cancers.[6] The proportion of breast cancer attributable to BRCA1 and BRCA2 increases with younger age of onset of the disease.

CANCER RISKS IN BRCA MUTATION CARRIERS

Carriers of mutations have a high life-time risk of breast cancer, with estimates of risk ranging from 65–85% for BRCA1 and 40–85% for BRCA2. There is also a high life-time risk of ovarian cancer estimated as 40–50% for BRCA1 and 10–25% for BRCA2.

The risks of both contralateral breast cancer and multiple ipsilateral primaries are also higher than that of the average breast cancer patient.[7] Risk of cancer at sites other than the breast and ovary is increased for both BRCA1 and BRCA2 mutation carriers, but to a lesser extent. BRCA1 carriers are at increased risk of cancers of the pancreas, stomach, fallopian tube, uterine body, cervix and prostate.[8] BRCA2 mutation carriers have been shown to have an increased risk of prostate, pancreatic, stomach, gallbladder and bile duct cancers, and malignant melanoma.[9] Male BRCA1 and BRCA2 carriers have an approximate 6% life-time risk of developing breast cancer, a 60–100-fold greater than that of men in the general population.[10,11]

Key point 1

- BRCA1 and BRCA2 gene mutation carriers are at high risk of developing breast and/or ovarian cancer.

CLINICAL ASPECTS OF BRCA-ASSOCIATED BREAST CANCER

BRCA1-associated breast cancer is mostly adenocarcinoma of the invasive ductal type.[12] An excess of medullary forms has been reported.[13] Frequently, cancers are of high grade and are oestrogen receptor, progesterone receptor, and HER-2 negative.[12,13] The pathological features suggest that breast cancer in women with a defective BRCA1 gene is more aggressive with evidence of a worse outcome than women with sporadic cancers. BRCA2-associated breast cancer is also generally invasive ductal of high histological grade, but does not have a clear association with hormone receptor status.

OTHER BREAST CANCER PREDISPOSITION GENES

Twin studies show that a quarter of breast cancer has an inherited component.[14] Furthermore, family history remains a predictive risk factor for breast cancer among non-carriers of BRCA1/2 mutations[15] and additional breast cancer susceptibility genes must, therefore, exist that contribute to

Table 1 Main hereditary breast cancer genes

Genes (name of syndrome)	Proportion of all breast cancer	Proportion of hereditary breast cancer associated with germline mutation	Breast cancer penetrance	Main other features of syndrome
BRCA1 (hereditary breast and ovarian cancer)	< 5%	10–20%	65–85% by age 70	Cancer of the ovary, pancreas, and prostate
BRCA2 (hereditary breast and ovarian cancer)	< 5%	10–20%	40–85% by age 70	Male breast cancer, cancer of the ovary, pancreas, and prostate
TP53 (Li-Fraumeni)	< 1%	< 1%	50% by age 50	Childhood sarcomas, brain tumours, leukaemia, lymphoma, adrenal cortical carcinoma
PTEN (Cowden)	< 1 in 1000	< 1%	30–50% by age 50	Hamartomas of skin and gastro-intestinal tract, benign and malignant thyroid tumours
STK11/LKB1 (Peutz-Jeghers)	?< 1 in 1000	< 1%	55% by age 64	Pigmented spots lips, buccal mucosa, skin; hamartomatous polyps gastro-intestinal tract; small bowel cancer
ATM (ataxia telangiectasia)	?1–13%	?8–10%	30% by age 70	No associated syndrome in AT heterozygotes
CHEK2 1100delC allele	1%	5%	? >20% by age 80	No associated syndrome

All figures are approximate.

heritable susceptibility to breast cancer in perhaps 30–50% of high-risk families. A number of genetic syndromes are associated with high breast cancer risk. Together, these rare syndromes account for only a very small proportion of hereditary disease. Other gene variants or polymorphisms have been identified as responsible for breast cancer with low penetrance, such as the ataxia-telangiectasia mutated (*ATM*) gene,[16] and *CHEK2*.[17] The clinical features of the most important/best known of these additional susceptibility genes are shown in Table 1.

RISK ASSESSMENT

Taking a detailed family history is the necessary first step in investigating a possible inherited predisposition to breast cancer. Cancer pedigrees should include at least first- and second-degree relatives and, ideally, third-degree relatives where possible and relevant. Both the maternal and paternal family histories should be documented. The great majority of women with a family history of breast cancer do not fall into a high-risk group and do not develop breast cancer. The important features to look for in a family history are: age at onset, bilateral disease, male breast cancer, multiple cases in one side of the family, other related early-onset tumours (especially ovarian cancer), the number of unaffected individuals, and Jewish ancestry.

In England and Wales, The National Institute for Clinical Excellence (NICE) has published Clinical Guidelines where individuals are placed into one of three risk categories of developing breast cancer on the basis of their family history that reflect where their care is likely to be delivered:[18]

Table 2 High-risk breast cancer families

Breast cancer only families
- Four or more relatives with breast cancer at any age, at least one of which is a first-degree
- Three first- or second-degree relatives affected with breast cancer at younger than an average age of 60 years
- Two first- or one first- and one second-degree relatives affected by breast cancer at younger than an average age of 50 years

Families with ovarian cancer
- Two first- or second-degree relatives with breast cancer at younger than an average age of 60 years and one ovarian cancer at any age
- One ovarian cancer at any age and one first-degree relative (may include that with ovarian cancer) or second-degree relative with breast cancer under age 50 years
- Two ovarian cancers at any age

Families with bilateral breast cancer
- One first- or second-degree relative with bilateral breast cancer and one first- or second-degree relative with breast cancer under 60 years
- One first-degree relative with bilateral breast cancer at younger than average age of 50 years

Families with male breast cancer
- Two first- or second-degree relatives with breast cancer at younger than an average age of 60 years and a male relative with breast cancer at any age
- One first- or second-degree relative with breast cancer under 50 and a male relative with breast cancer at any age

Definition of high risk:	risk > 8% between ages 40–50 years or a life-time risk of ≥ 30%, or ≥ 20% chance of *BRCA1/2* or *TP53* mutation.
First-degree relatives:	mother, father, daughter, son, sister, brother.
Second-degree relatives:	grandparents, grandchildren, aunt, uncle, niece and nephew, half-sister, half-brother.

1. **Near population risk**, *i.e.* 10-year risk of < 3% between ages 40–50 years and a life-time risk of < 17% are cared for in primary care (general practice).

2. **Moderate risk**, *i.e.* 10-year risk of 3–8% between ages 40–50 years or a life-time risk between 17–30% are cared for in secondary care (breast units).

3. **High risk**, *i.e.* 10-year risk of > 8% between ages 40–50 years, or a life-time risk ≥ 30%, or a ≥ 20% chance of a faulty *BRCA1/2* gene in the family are cared for in tertiary care (clinical genetics and specialist services).

Key point 2–4

- The great majority of women with a family history of breast cancer do not fall into a high-risk group and do not develop breast cancer.

- Taking a detailed family history is the first step in investigating a possible inherited predisposition to breast cancer.

- The important features to look for in a family history are: age at onset, bilateral disease, male breast cancer, multiple cases in one side of the family, ovarian cancer, and Jewish ancestry.

Examples of typical family histories falling in the high-risk group are given in Table 2.

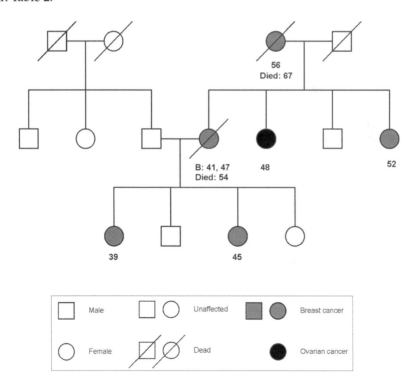

Fig. 1 Family tree of hereditary breast/ovarian cancer syndrome. Figures under symbols are age of cancer diagnosis or, when stated, age at death. B, bilateral cancer.

Many breast units in the UK have introduced Family History Clinics (FHCs), where the initial step of stratification of referrals into risk categories is taken, based on the family history information received. Individuals classified as at near population risk may be re-assured and managed in primary care. Only those individuals assessed as at moderate- or high-risk are usually seen at a FHC. Calculations of individualised breast cancer risk strata are made from the pedigree data. Those suggestive of hereditary cancer syndromes have salient features such as the examples shown in Figure 1.

Mathematical and computerised risk-assessment models have been introduced that permit risk calculations in terms of an age-specific risk (*e.g.* risk over the next 10 years), or as a life-time risk (e.g. risk to age 80 years). These constitute helpful aids to the manual clinical assessment of family trees, but have important limitations as to the accuracy of their risk estimates. Gaining popularity in the UK, the Manchester scoring system[19] predicts the probability of finding a *BRCA1/2* mutation by attributing a score to each cancer case in a family (scores vary according to the site and age of onset of the cancer) and relating the total score to likelihood of finding a mutation in an affected family member.

GENETIC TESTING

Outside certain populations (*e.g.* Ashkenazi Jews) with a few recurrent mutations, the search for mutations in the *BRCA* genes represents a daunting task; it is both time consuming and expensive, often requiring the combination of several technical approaches. Mutation screening needs, therefore, to be targeted to ensure a relatively high detection rate. NICE guidelines recommend that testing for breast cancer predisposition genes should be offered to women with a 20% or greater chance of carrying a mutation.[18] Genetic testing should only be carried out after informed consent is obtained. This should be preceded by in-depth genetic counselling including an explanation of the cancer risk, the benefits and limitations of testing, the far-reaching psychological and insurance-related implications, and the options for surveillance and risk reduction in those who test positive.

Key point 5

- Genetic mutation screening is carried out in an individual already affected by cancer.

GENETIC MUTATION SCREENING

In the first instance, genetic mutation screening is carried out in an individual already affected by cancer. In interpreting mutational analysis results, it is worth noting that even the gold standard technique, full gene sequencing, does not have a 100% detection rate. A negative mutation search may, therefore, not be a true negative. It may reflect the failure of the laboratory techniques to detect a genetic fault, or it may be that a mutation is present in another gene involved in familial breast cancer. When a mutation search is uninformative in high-risk families, the option of blood storage may allow for future analysis with novel techniques, or testing for new genes.

PREDICTIVE GENETIC TESTING

Predictive genetic testing, that is testing in individuals unaffected by cancer, may be carried out only after a mutation is identified in an affected member of the family. It is important, in this circumstance, to remind the person being tested that he/she has at most a 50% chance of carrying the same mutation as his/her affected relative. If a mutation is found at predictive testing then that individual has a high risk of developing breast and/or ovarian cancer. If a mutation in the family is established and an unaffected family member tests negative for that mutation, his/her test result can be regarded as true negative. However, a recent study suggests that the breast/ovarian cancer risk may still remain higher than that of the general population, perhaps equivalent to that of a woman in the moderate-risk category.[20]

Of the seven genes presented in Table 1, *BRCA1* and *BRCA2* are the most commonly tested and *BRCA* mutations explain a considerable proportion of the very high-risk families, particularly if ovarian or male breast cancer is present. Mutations in *TP53* and *PTEN* genes are significantly rarer. *TP53* mutations are usually identified in families with Li-Fraumeni syndrome-associated tumours, and *PTEN* mutations are found in families with Cowden's syndrome. Clinical genetic testing for *ATM*, *STK11* and *CHEK2* genes has not been implemented.

Key point 6

- Predictive genetic testing, that is testing in individuals unaffected by cancer, may be carried out only after a mutation is identified in an affected member of the family.

RISK-REDUCING STRATEGIES

Four options are currently available to reduce breast cancer incidence in women at increased risk – early detection, chemoprevention, risk-reducing surgery, and life-style advice.

EARLY DETECTION

Mammography

The mainstay of early detection is regular screening of the breasts by mammography. In the general population, the balance between benefits and harms of screening women aged 40–49 years is unclear. One reason for this is thought to be the decreased incidence of breast cancer at younger age. A 50-year-old woman, without a significant family history, entering the UK National Health Service Breast Screening Programme (NHSBSP) has a 10-year risk estimate of developing breast cancer of 2.8% and a life-time risk (to age 80 years) of around 17%.[1] A woman in the moderate- or high-risk category has at least the same level of breast cancer risk at age 40 years, which from an incidence viewpoint alone suggests that mammographic screening from age 40 years may be worthwhile.

However, several other factors need to be considered when evaluating the benefit/risk ratio of screening mammography for young women with familial breast cancer, namely: (i) the decreased sensitivity of mammography at younger age in general;[21] (ii) its lower sensitivity in *BRCA* carriers;[22] (iii) concern about the increased cancer risk from early radiation exposure; (iv) poorer compliance in younger women; (v) unknown cost-effectiveness; and (vi) potential psychological distress. Pooled data from 22 UK breast units offering screening to women under 50 years of age with a significant family history of breast cancer has shown rates of cancer detection and incidence similar to those of the NHSBSP for women aged 50–64 years.[23] The evidence from this and other studies suggests that screening mammography for young women with familial breast cancer risk may be effective, and lead to a survival benefit. As there is unlikely to be a sufficiently large, randomised, controlled trial to prove this, there is currently in the UK an on-going Health Technology Assessment of mammographic screening in this group of women (FH01) to assess the efficacy of screening mammography. NICE guidelines recommend annual mammographic surveillance for women aged 40–49 years at moderate- and high-risk. Digital mammography, when available, should be used in preference to conventional film mammography as it provides better resolution, especially in dense breast tissue of younger women. Screening for women aged 30–39 years and more frequent screening for those aged 50 years or older is only recommended as part of a research or audit study. Mammography for women younger than 30 years is not recommended.[18,24]

Key point 7

- Mammographic screening is currently the surveillance method most widely used for high risk women, but MRI screening is now recommended in gene mutation carriers.

Magnetic resonance imaging (MRI)

Four large observational studies of screening MRI in high-risk women have now been published. The MARIBS study in the UK detected 35 cancers in 649 women aged 35–49 years with a strong family history of breast cancer, including 120 *BRCA* carriers.[25] MRI was more than twice as sensitive as mammography (77% versus 40%) at the expense of lower specificity (81% versus 93%). The improved sensitivity was more pronounced in the subgroup of *BRCA1* carriers, where MRI detected 92% of tumours whereas mammography only detected 23%. MRI studies in The Netherlands,[26] Canada[27] and Germany[28] have shown a similar improvement in sensitivity, but lower specificity compared to mammography.

Current NICE guidelines recommend that annual MRI surveillance should be offered, in addition to mammography, to women aged 40–49 years at a 10-year risk > 20%, or risk > 12% if they have a dense breast pattern on mammography. For women aged 30–39 years, MRI surveillance can be offered to women at a 10-year year risk of > 8%. *BRCA1/2* carriers aged 30–49 years and *TP53* mutation carriers aged ≥ 20 years may also be offered annual MRI.[24]

CHEMOPREVENTION

Tamoxifen

Tamoxifen has been proposed as a potential chemopreventative agent in women at increased risk. The main rationale for this is the finding of a reduced incidence of contralateral breast cancers in randomised trials of tamoxifen usage in breast cancer patients. Tamoxifen is a synthetic drug that acts as a selective oestrogen receptor modulator, *i.e.* has functionally mixed partial agonist and antagonist properties of the natural hormone.

Four randomised controlled trials have reported inconsistent results as to the effect of tamoxifen in breast cancer prevention. Smaller UK[29] and Italian[30] studies failed to detect a difference in breast cancer incidence between the tamoxifen and placebo groups. The largest North American NSABP-P1 study[31] reported a 49% reduction of invasive breast cancer with tamoxifen. The International Breast Intervention Study 1 (IBIS 1)[32] showed a 32% risk reduction with tamoxifen in women at increased risk of breast cancer. This and the NSABP-P1 study showed a 2-fold increase in endometrial cancers and venous thrombo-embolism in the tamoxifen group.

Key point 8

- Chemoprevention trials of tamoxifen have shown a significant breast cancer risk reduction in women at increased risk, but also an increase in the risks of thrombo-embolic events and endometrial cancer.

Tamoxifen is not currently licensed in the UK for use as a primary chemo-prevention agent and its wide use to that effect cannot be recommended.

Raloxifene

More selective anti-oestrogens with less toxic effects than tamoxifen have been looked at. The Study of Tamoxifen and Raloxifene (STAR) compared tamoxifen 20 mg/day versus raloxifene 60 mg/day in nearly 20,000 women at high risk of developing breast cancer. After a median follow-up of 4 years, both drugs reduced the relative risk for breast cancer by about 50%, with fewer cases of endometrial cancer and fewer thrombo-embolic events in the raloxifene group.[33]

Aromatase inhibitors

Inhibitors of the aromatase enzyme have been shown to be more effective than tamoxifen in preventing tumour recurrence and contralateral disease in postmenopausal women previously treated for breast cancer, without the increase of endometrial cancer or venous thrombo-embolism.[34] The use of an aromatase inhibitor (anastrozole) for primary chemoprevention is being evaluated in the second International Breast Cancer Intervention Study (IBIS II).

RISK-REDUCING SURGERY

Bilateral risk-reducing mastectomy (BRRM)

Bilateral mastectomy is an option available to women at increased risk of breast cancer due to a family history of the disease. Surgery aims to remove the majority of the 'at-risk' breast tissue with a corresponding reduction in cancer risk. Data from several major observational studies[35–37] represent the best available evidence of the efficacy of BRRM in reducing breast cancer incidence by around 90%, especially in high-risk carriers of *BRCA* mutations.

It is important to remember that BRRM will not prevent the development of all breast cancers. Case reports have reported the subsequent development of breast cancer in women after both total and subcutaneous mastectomy. A subcutaneous mastectomy leaves behind the nipple and areola complex with a variable proportion of the major subareolar duct system. With a simple mastectomy, more breast tissue is likely to be removed, as an ellipse of skin and the nipple-areola complex are removed and better access is achieved to the superior aspect of the breast. However, some breast tissue will remain below the skin flaps regardless of the skill of the surgeon. Although suspected, no clear evidence exists from the above or other studies that total mastectomy is more effective than subcutaneous mastectomy in reducing the incidence of breast cancer. A third technique, skin-sparing mastectomy, removes the nipple and areola but preserves a very thin flap of skin over the remainder of the breast; this may enhance the cosmetic result compared with simple mastectomy, and its efficacy should be intermediate between that of simple and subcutaneous mastectomy.

In a clinical setting, there is a high demand for *BRCA1/2* testing and for risk reducing surgery (both mastectomy and oophorectomy) by women from high-risk families. Attitudes towards BRRM vary widely, with some women and their physicians considering this an unacceptable intervention. A small proportion of women do subsequently regret their decision to proceed with BRRM, and this is more likely if the option was raised by a clinician rather than themselves. In some centres, pre-operative psychological assessment is used to identify those women who may subsequently regret choosing surgery.

BRRM is appropriate only for a small proportion of women who are from high-risk families and should ideally be managed by a multidisciplinary team. Women considering BRRM should have genetic counselling in a specialist cancer genetics clinic before a decision is made. Discussion of individual breast cancer risk and its potential reduction by surgery should take into account individual risk factors and include the woman's current age – especially at extremes of age ranges. At BRRM, some women are found to have breast cancer histologically, and this possibility should be discussed pre-operatively. Women considering BRRM should have the opportunity to discuss their breast reconstruction options, immediate and delayed, with a member of a surgical team with specialist oncoplastic or breast-reconstructive skills. BRRM does not have a detrimental impact on body image or sexual dysfunction for the majority of women although for some women it is associated with adverse psychosocial effects such as emotional instability, stress, and low self-esteem.

The decision to undergo BRRM is an individual one. In general, BRRM should be presented in a non-directive fashion to *BRCA1/2* carriers and it may also be a reasonable option for women of equivalent high risk where predictive genetic testing is not possible; whenever a gene mutation is not identified, family history details should be verified before surgery. It should not be performed in women whose family history is not suggestive of an inherited factor even if anxiety about breast cancer is high.

Key point 9

- Risk reducing surgery (mastectomy and oophorectomy) can significantly reduce breast cancer risk.

Bilateral risk-reducing oophorectomy (BRRO)

Several observational studies provide evidence that BRRO reduces breast, ovarian and *BRCA*-related gynaecological cancer (coelomic epithelial cancer) in high-risk women.[38,39] These show an approximate 50% pre-menopausal breast cancer risk reduction and 90% reduction in ovarian cancer risk. Although the penetrance of ovarian cancer is lower than that of breast cancer in *BRCA1/2* carriers (25–50% life-time risk), the absence of reliable methods of early detection and the lethality of advanced ovarian cancer have prompted many oncologists to recommend BRRO after childbearing is complete. The primary negative effect of BRRO in pre-menopausal women is the induction of premature menopause.

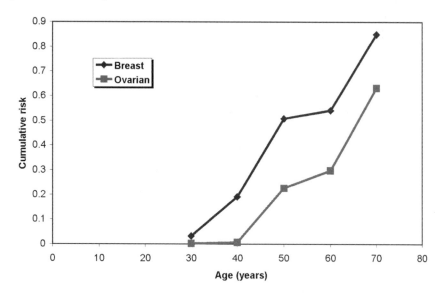

Fig. 2 Cumulative risk of breast and ovarian cancer in *BRCA1* mutation carriers with age.

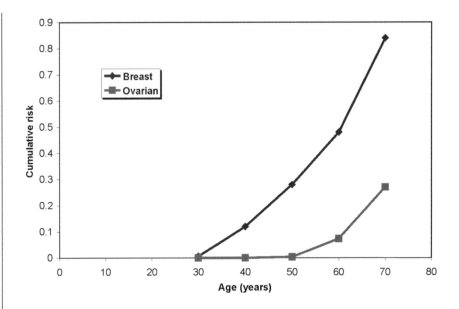

Fig. 3 Cumulative risk of breast and ovarian cancer in *BRCA2* mutation carriers with age.

Breast cancer risk for *BRCA1/2* carriers rises most dramatically when a woman is in her 40s and the rise is steeper for *BRCA1*. Ovarian carcinoma risk rises later and in parallel to breast cancer risk for both *BRCA1* and *BRCA2* carriers (Figs 2 and 3).[5,40] The average age at diagnosis for *BRCA2*-associated ovarian cancers is similar to that for sporadic cancers, whereas that for *BRCA1*-associated ovarian cancer is about 10 years younger. Therefore, theoretically, prophylactic surgery could be delayed by 5–10 years for *BRCA2* carriers; delaying BRRO until the completion of childbearing in the mid-40s delays also the induction of premature menopause and avoids, to some extent, potential concerns of whether to administer hormone replacement therapy (HRT) or not.

Since tumours can arise from the fallopian tubes in *BRCA1/2* carriers, BRRO should include complete removal of the tubes as well as the ovaries. Laparoscopic surgery is now the method of choice for BRRO unless there are contra-indications.

Key point 10

- Risk-reducing surgery is appropriate only for a small proportion of women from high-risk families and should be managed by a multidisciplinary team.

LIFE-STYLE ADVICE

Environmental and life-style factors, rather than inherited factors, account for most cases of the inter-individual differences in breast cancer susceptibility. It is important to convey information to individuals at increased familial risk about factors which are modifiable and where behavioural changes may reduce the risk of developing breast cancer. This should include advice on HRT and hormonal contraceptive usage, family planning and breast-feeding, weight and physical activity, alcohol consumption, *etc.*[18]

SCREENING FOR OTHER CANCERS

OVARIAN CANCER

The traditional screening methods for ovarian carcinoma are measurement of the tumour marker CA 125, transvaginal ultrasonography, and clinical pelvic examination. The available evidence does not justify ovarian screening in the general population. For women at risk of hereditary ovarian cancer, the appropriate screening strategy remains undefined and the UK Cancer Family Study Group recommends ovarian screening to be offered only as part of clinical trials; outcome data are being collected as part of a national study.

CONCLUSIONS

Women at hereditary risk of breast cancer face a difficult and complicated clinical decision, in terms of trade-offs. Each of the options available to them

Table 3 Management options for women at high risk of developing breast cancer

Modality	Advantages	Disadvantages
Surveillance (mammography MRI)	Non-invasive Detects disease early MRI may be useful in *BRCA* carriers	Does not prevent disease Poor sensitivity of mammography in *BRCA* carriers Unknown effect on mortality reduction Adherence unknown
Tamoxifen	Decreases risk of breast cancer by a third Possible larger effect in *BRCA2* mutation carriers	Effect on oestrogen-positive tumours only Doubles the risk of thrombo-embolic events and endometrial cancer Duration of benefit unknown Overall risk/benefit ratio unclear
Prophylactic oophorectomy	50% breast cancer risk reduction (including *BRCA* carriers) in pre-menopausal women	Premature menopause, with cardiovascular and skeletal side effects Impact of long-term HRT on risk reduction in young *BRCA* carriers unknown Psychosexual outcomes unknown
Prophylactic mastectomy	90% breast cancer risk reduction (including *BRCA* carriers) High satisfaction levels	Major surgery, with reconstructive procedures and potential for complications

has unique advantages and disadvantages that are summarised in Table 3. It is vital that women at high risk have access to a genetic counsellor that can encourage them to take time to understand both their risk level and the advantages and disadvantages of the options before them.

Key points for clinical practice

- *BRCA1* and *BRCA2* gene mutation carriers are at high risk of developing breast and/or ovarian cancer.

- Taking a detailed family history is the first step in investigating a possible inherited predisposition to breast cancer.

- The great majority of women with a family history of breast cancer do not fall into a high-risk group and do not develop breast cancer.

- The important features to look for in a family history are: age at onset, bilateral disease, male breast cancer, multiple cases in one side of the family, ovarian cancer, and Jewish ancestry.

- Genetic mutation screening is carried out in an individual already affected by cancer.

- Predictive genetic testing, that is testing in individuals unaffected by cancer, may be carried out only after a mutation is identified in an affected member of the family.

- Mammographic screening is currently the surveillance method most widely used for high risk women, but MRI screening is now recommended in gene mutation carriers.

- Chemoprevention trials of tamoxifen have shown a significant breast cancer risk reduction in women at increased risk, but also an increase in the risks of thrombo-embolic events and endometrial cancer.

- Risk reducing surgery (mastectomy and oophorectomy) can significantly reduce breast cancer risk.

- Risk-reducing surgery is appropriate only for a small proportion of women from high-risk families and should be managed by a multidisciplinary team.

References

1. Toms JR. (ed) *CancerStats Monograph*. London: Cancer Research UK, 2004.
2. Collaborative Group on Hormonal Factors in Breast Cancer. Familial breast cancer: collaborative reanalysis of individual data from 52 epidemiological studies including 58 209 women with breast cancer and 101 986 women without the disease. *Lancet* 2001; **358**: 1389–1399.
3. Claus EB, Schildkraut JM, Thompson WD, Risch NJ. The genetic attributable risk of breast and ovarian cancer. *Cancer* 1996; **76**: 2318–2324.
4. Easton DF, Bishop DT, Ford D, Crockford GP, Breast Cancer Linkage Consortium. Genetic linkage analysis in familial breast and ovarian cancer: results from 214 families. *Am J Hum Genet* 1993; **52**: 678–707.

5. Ford D, Easton DF, Stratton M *et al.* Genetic heterogeneity and penetrance analysis of the *BRCA1* and *BRCA2* genes in breast cancer families. *Am J Hum Genet* 1998; **62**: 676–689.

6. Warner E, Foulkes W, Goodwin P *et al.* Prevalence and penetrance of *BRCA1* and *BRCA2* gene mutations in unselected Ashkenazi Jewish women with breast cancer. *J Natl Cancer Inst* 1999; **91**: 1241–1247.

7. Metcalfe K, Lynch HT, Ghadirian P *et al.* Contralateral breast cancer in *BRCA1* and *BRCA2* mutation carriers. *J Clin Oncol* 2004; **22**: 2328–2335.

8. Thompson D, Easton DF, Breast Cancer Linkage Consortium. Cancer incidence in BRCA1 mutation carriers. *J Natl Cancer Inst* 2002; **94**: 1358–1365.

9. Breast Cancer Linkage Consortium. Cancer risks in *BRCA2* mutation carriers. *J Natl Cancer Inst* 1999; **91**: 1316.

10. Brose MS, Rebbeck TR, Calzone KA *et al.* Cancer risk estimates for *BRCA1* mutation carriers identified in a risk evaluation program. *J Natl Cancer Inst* 2002; **94**: 1365–1372.

11. Thompson D, Easton D, Breast Cancer Linkage Consortium. Variation in cancer risks, by mutation position, in *BRCA2* mutation carriers. *Am J Hum Genet* 2001; **68**: 410–419.

12. Breast Cancer Linkage Consortium. Pathology of familial breast cancer: differences between breast cancers in carriers of *BRCA1* and *BRCA2* mutations and sporadic cases. *Lancet* 1997; **349**: 1505–1510.

13. Eisinger F, Nogues C, Guinebretiere JM *et al.* Novel indications for *BRCA1* screening using individual clinical and morphological features. *Int J Cancer* 1999; **84**: 263–267.

14. Lichtenstein P, Holm NV, Verkasalo PK *et al.* Environmental and heritable factors in the causation of cancer. *N Engl J Med* 2000; **343**: 78–85.

15. Claus EB, Schildkraut J, Iversen Jr ES, Berry D, Parmigiani G. Effect of *BRCA1* and *BRCA2* on the association between breast cancer risk and family history. *J Natl Cancer Inst* 1998; **90**: 1824–1829.

16. Easton DF. Cancer risks in A-T heterozygotes. *Int J Radiat Biol* 1994; **66**: S177–S182.

17. CHEK2-Breast Cancer Consortium. Low-penetrance susceptibility to breast cancer due to CHEK2*1100delC in noncarriers of *BRCA1* or *BRCA2* mutations. *Nat Genet* 2002; **31**: 55–59.

18. McIntosh A, Shaw C, Evans G *et al. Clinical guidelines and evidence review of the classification and care of women at risk of familial breast cancer.* London: National Collaborating Centre for Primary Care/University of Sheffield, 2004.

19. Evans DGR, Lalloo F, Wallace A, Rahman N. Update on the Manchester Scoring System for *BRCA1* and *BRCA2* testing. *J Med Genet* 2005; **42**: e39.

20. Smith A, Moran A, Boyd MC *et al.* Phenocopies in *BRCA1* and *BRCA2* families: evidence for modifier genes and implications for screening *J Med Genet* 2007; 4: 10–15.

21. Sibbering DM, Burrell HC, Evans AJ *et al.* Mammographic sensitivity in women under 50 years presenting symptomatically with breast cancer. *Breast* 1995; **4**: 127–129.

22. Goffin J, Chappuis PO, Wong N, Foulkes WD. Re: Magnetic resonance imaging and mammography in women with a hereditary risk of breast cancer [letter]. *J Natl Cancer Inst* 2001; **93**: 1754–1755.

23. Macmillan RD. Screening women with a family history of breast cancer – results from the British Familial Breast Cancer Group. *Eur J Surg Oncol* 2000; **26**: 149–152.

24. National Institute for Health and Clinical Excellence. *Familial breast cancer: the classification and care of women at risk of familial breast cancer in primary, secondary and tertiary care.* NICE clinical guideline 41. London: Department of Health, 2006.

25. Leach MO, Boggis CR, Dixon AK *et al.* Screening with magnetic resonance imaging and mammography of a UK population at high familial risk of breast cancer: a prospective multicentre cohort study (MARIBS). *Lancet* 2005; **365**: 1769–1778.

26. Kriege M, Brekelmans CTM, Boetes C *et al.* Efficacy of MRI and mammography for breast-cancer screening in women with a familial or genetic predisposition. *N Engl J Med* 2004; **351**: 427–437.

27. Warner E, Causer PA. MRI surveillance for hereditary breast-cancer risk. *Lancet* 2005; **365**: 1747–1748.

28. Kuhl CK, Schrading S, Leutner CC *et al.* Mammography, breast ultrasound, and magnetic resonance imaging for surveillance of women at high familial risk for breast cancer. *J Clin Oncol* 2005; **23**: 8469–8476.

29. Powles T, Eeles R, Asheley S *et al.* Interim analysis of the incidence of breast cancer in

the Royal Marsden Hospital tamoxifen randomised chemoprevention trial. *Lancet* 1998; **352**: 98–101.

30. Veronesi U, Maisonneuve P, Sacchini V *et al*. Prevention of breast cancer with tamoxifen: preliminary findings from the Italian randomised trial among hysterectomised women. *Lancet* 1998; **352**: 93–97.

31. Fisher B, Costantino JP, Wickerham DL *et al*. Tamoxifen for prevention of breast cancer: report of the National Surgical Adjuvant Breast and Bowel Project P1 Study. *J Natl Cancer Inst* 1998; **90**: 1371–1388.

32. IBIS Investigators. First results from the International Breast Cancer Intervention Study (IBIS-I): a randomised prevention trial. *Lancet* 2002; **360**: 817–824.

33. Vogel VG, Costantino JP, Wickerham DL *et al*. Effects of tamoxifen vs. raloxifene on the risk of developing invasive breast cancer and other disease outcomes: the NSABP Study of Tamoxifen and Raloxifene (STAR) P-2 Trial. *JAMA* 2006; **295**: 2727–2741.

34. Baum M, Buzdar A, Cuzick J *et al*. Anastrozole alone or in combination with tamoxifen versus tamoxifen alone for adjuvant treatment of postmenopausal women with early-stage breast cancer: results of the ATAC (Arimidex, Tamoxifen Alone or in Combination) trial efficacy and safety update analysis. *Cancer* 2003; **98**: 1802–1810.

35. Hartmann LC, Sellers TA, Schaid DJ *et al*. Efficacy of bilateral prophylactic mastectomy in *BRCA1* and *BRCA2* gene mutation carriers. *J Natl Cancer Inst* 2001; **93**: 1633–1637.

36. Rebbeck TR, Friebel T, Lynch HT *et al*. Bilateral prophylactic mastectomy reduces breast cancer risk in BRCA1 and BRCA2 mutation carriers: the PROSE Study Group. *J Clin Oncol* 2004; **22**: 1055–1062.

37. Meijers-Heijboer H, van Geel B, van Putten WLJ *et al*. Breast cancer after prophylactic bilateral mastectomy in women with a *BRCA1* or *BRCA2* mutation. *N Engl J Med* 2001; **345**: 159–164.

38. Rebbeck TR, Lynch HT, Neuhausen SL *et al*. Prophylactic oophorectomy in carriers of *BRCA1* or *BRCA2* mutations. *N Engl J Med* 2002; **346**: 1616–1622.

39. Kauff ND, Domchek SM, Friebel TM *et al*. Multi-center prospective analysis of risk-reducing salpingo-oophorectomy to prevent BRCA-associated breast and ovarian cancer. 2006. Proceedings from the 42nd annual meeting of the American Society of Clinical Oncology. Atlanta, GA. Abstract 1003.

40. Easton DF, Bishop DT, Ford D, Breast Cancer Linkage Consortium. Breast and ovarian cancer incidence in BRCA1-mutation carriers. *Am J Hum Genet* 1995; **56**: 265–271.

Eva M. Weiler-Mithoff

7

Latissimus dorsi flap in breast reconstruction

Breast reconstruction can help a woman to feel whole again, re-establishes body symmetry and plays a significant role in the woman's physical, emotional and psychological recovery from breast cancer.[1]

The current aim of breast reconstruction is to match the remaining breast in terms of contour, dimension and position.[2] Immediate breast reconstruction (IBR) is cost effective and allows maximum preservation of breast skin and preservation of the inframammary fold. Skin sparing mastectomy in particular facilitates better cosmetic results with a reduced need for balancing surgery.[3,4] IBR does not adversely affect breast cancer outcome and does not interfere with further treatment even for advanced cancers but may improve the overall outlook, psychological rehabilitation and quality of remaining life.[1,5–9] Chemotherapy and radiotherapy may have detrimental effects on some types of immediate breast reconstruction. These can be avoided by judicious choice of type and timing of reconstructive techniques.[10]

Key point 1 & 2

- Breast reconstruction plays a significant role in the woman's physical, emotional and psychological recovery from breast cancer.

- The ideal breast reconstruction is a soft, natural-feeling breast which maintains its characteristics over time as a natural ptosis or droop and a permanent and natural inframammary fold.

Eva M. Weiler-Mithoff FRCS(Ed.) FRCS(Glasg) Plast
Consultant Plastic and Reconstructive Surgeon, Canniesburn Unit, Jubilee Building, Glasgow Royal Infirmary, 84 Castle Street, Glasgow G4 0SF, UK
E-mail: eva.weiler-mithoff@northglasgow.scot.nhs.uk

Delayed breast reconstruction requires replacement of a larger amount of breast skin and avoids the detrimental affects of radiotherapy on the reconstruction but the mastectomy flaps may be scarred and suffer from the effects of radiotherapy. The end result of the breast reconstruction may, therefore, not be as aesthetically pleasing.

In the age of limited financial resources, targets and deadlines, it is even more important to select a range of techniques which are most cost-effective, have low revision rates, a low rate of symmetry surgery and are able to withstand adjuvant radiotherapy. The latissimus dorsi flap is such a highly versatile technique and has acceptable donor site morbidity. It can serve as an ideal reconstructive technique for the majority of patients.

Traditionally the latissimus dorsi flap has been used to cover a breast implant if the patient was not suitable for an implant reconstruction alone or an abdominal flap. The implant-based techniques allow some patient control over breast size, but the quality of the long-term result is directly related to the tolerance of breast implants. Further procedures are required for complications and maintenance. The aesthetic results from totally autologous latissimus dorsi reconstructions are superior to latissimus dorsi flaps with implants due to their more natural appearance, consistency and durability. Autologous tissue can also better withstand radiotherapy.[11]

Key point 3 & 4

- Immediate breast reconstruction is safe, has no known oncological disadvantages, is most cost-effective and leads to the best cosmetic results due to maximum preservation of breast skin but exposes the reconstructions to the effects of radiotherapy.

- Delayed reconstruction involves a separate episode of hospitalisation, requires replacement of a larger amount of skin and potentially poor mastectomy flaps.

ANATOMY

The latissimus dorsi muscle is a large triangular back muscle of variable thickness. It arises from the thoracolumbar fascia, the spinous processes of the thoracic, lumbar and sacral vertebrae, the posterior part of iliac crest, the lower 3–4 ribs and the tip of the scapula. The muscle inserts with a tendon into the inter-tubercular groove of humerus. The main vascular supply is through the thoracodorsal vessels, the terminal branch of the sub-scapular axis. Additional blood supply is received through the serratus branch which is able to perfuse the latissimus dorsi muscle retrogradely through connections to the lateral thoracic vessels even if the main thoracodorsal pedicle has been divided.[12] Segmental branches from intercostal vessels and para-spinal perforators provide the main blood supply to the distal portion of the flap and are the vascular basis of a distally pedicled latissimus dorsi flap. This technique has been used for the cover of spina bifida or lumbar defects of other aetiology. The latissimus dorsi muscle is classed as a Type V muscle according to Mathes and

Nahai.[13] Nerve supply to the muscle is through the thoracodorsal nerve which arises from C6–8. This nerve is thought to contain mainly motor fibres. The sensation to the skin overlying the muscle is provided by segmental sensory skin branches.

The cutaneous territory of this flap consists of the skin superficial to the entire muscle and about 3 cm beyond –about 30 cm x 40 cm. Numerous myocutaneous perforators allow the design of skin islands in various patterns but orientation of the skin paddle in the relaxed skin tension lines allows maximum skin harvest with a good scar, which can be hidden under the bra strap.

LATISSIMUS DORSI FLAP WITH IMPLANT

The latissimus dorsi flap was originally described at the turn of the last century by Tansini, an Italian surgeon, for the closure of the radical mastectomy defect. Unfortunately, the significance of this technique was not realised at that time, soon forgotten and only rediscovered 75 years later independently by Olivari, Muehlbauer and McCraw.[14–17] Schneider described the surgical anatomy of the latissimus dorsi muscle in detail and realised the potential of this flap not only for chest wall resurfacing but also for breast reconstruction.[18] McCraw, Bostwick and Maxwell published the first clinical series using the latissimus dorsi muscle to provide vascularity to the skin-island and protection of the underlying silicone implant. The latissimus dorsi flap with implant became the standard method of breast reconstruction in the 1970s, allowing the reconstruction of larger more pendulous breasts (Figs 1A,B and 2A–D).[19] Its popularity was lost due to the extremely high incidence of implant complications. After the introduction of the transverse rectus abdominis myocutaneous (TRAM) flap in 1979, which offered a completely autologous breast reconstruction, the classical latissimus dorsi flap with implant was

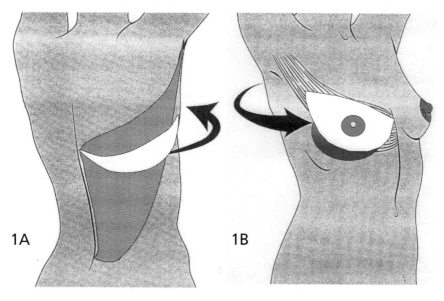

1A

1B

Fig. 1 (A,B) Classical latissimus dorsi myocutaneous flap and implant breast reconstruction.

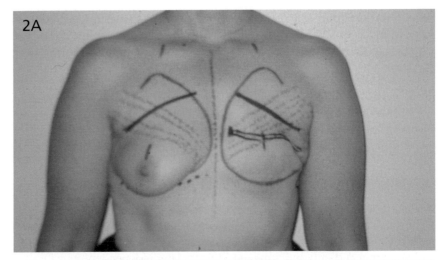

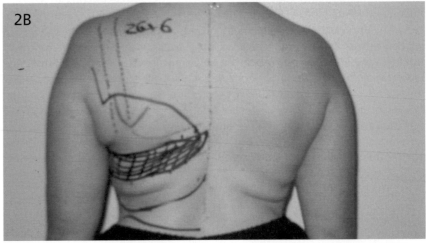

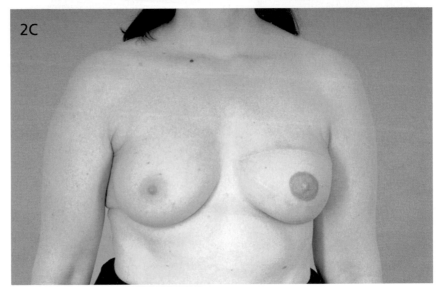

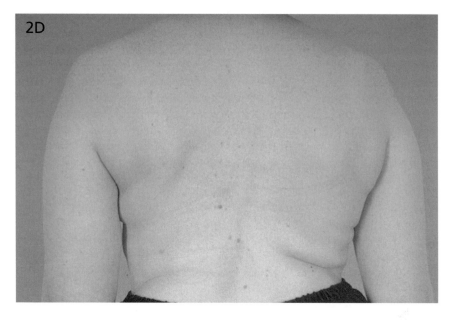

Fig. 2 Delayed breast reconstruction latissimus dorsi flap and implant, augmentation of contralateral breast. (A,B) Preoperative views; (C,D) Postoperative views.

relegated to cases which were not suitable for implant-only reconstructions or TRAM flaps.

AUTOLOGOUS LATISSIMUS DORSI FLAP

Ever since the early 1980s, surgeons tried to modify the latissimus dorsi flap harvest in order to increase the volume of the flap and avoid the use of a breast implant. Boehme and Papp described the buried, de-epithelialised latissimus dorsi flap, Hokin used an extended, oblique skin paddle together with the entire muscle and lumbar fascia and Marshall published a T-shaped skin paddle which was partially de-epithelialised. All these types of autologous or extended latissimus dorsi flap were rarely used due to significant problems caused by too extensive soft tissue harvest and poor donor site cosmesis.[20–23] McCraw and Papp were the first to harvest additional soft tissue in the form of a thin layer of fat on the surface of the latissimus dorsi muscle, the scapular area and the so-called supra iliac fat pad. Their *fleur-de-lys* skin island design was later abandoned due to poor healing of the donor site.[24] Barnett's added fat flap increased the flap volume by harvesting a 5-cm cuff of full-thickness subcutaneous tissue surrounding the skin island, but this also resulted in bad contour and delayed wound healing on the back.[25]

Germann and Steinau eventually described the parascapular extension, an adipofascial flap overlying the scapula and perfused by perforators from the cranial edge of the latissimus dorsi muscle.[26] This allowed a substantial increase in flap volume without obvious contour deformity. The most recent and most reliable modification of the extended or autologous latissimus dorsi flap was described by Delay and colleagues in 1998 (Fig. 3A,B).[27] They managed to double the flap volume by harvesting a large skin island, the entire

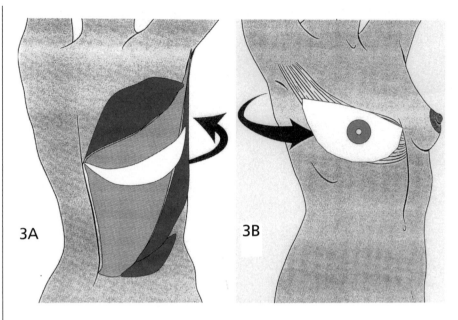

Fig. 3 (A,B) Extended autologous latissimus dorsi flap.

muscle and subcutaneous fat tissue from six areas of additional fat harvest at the level of or below Scarpa's fascia. The additional areas of fat harvest were: (i) fat under skin island; (ii) fat overlying surface of muscle; (iii) parascapular adipofascial extension; (iv) fat anterior to muscle; (v) supra-iliac 'love handles'; and (vi) fat underneath muscle.

Several large series of this type of autologous latissimus dorsi flap have since been published and this extremely reliable and versatile technique has now started to revolutionise immediate breast reconstruction because it offers a completely autologous reconstruction, avoids all implant-related complications and has acceptable donor site function and cosmesis.[28,29] Most importantly, this technique can be used in immediate breast reconstruction when the need for adjuvant radiotherapy may only become obvious after surgery.

ADVANTAGES AND DISADVANTAGES

Latissimus dorsi flap breast reconstruction is a very versatile, safe and reliable technique with a success rate of over 99%. Like abdominal tissue reconstruction, it is able to provide a completely autologous reconstruction but avoids rectus muscle harvest and the complications of free tissue transfers. This technique is, therefore, suitable even for high-risk patients. Disadvantages include a donor scar on the back which can be avoided by use of endoscopic techniques. The colour match of back and breast skin may not be ideal and there may be a limit to the amount of skin and soft tissue which can be transferred. An additional abdominal advancement flap may be required in order to replace a larger amount of breast skin. Alternatively, the breast skin can be pre-expanded or the breast skin flaps can be held out to length by initial insertion of a tissue expander after skin sparing mastectomy. If there is not enough bulk on the back for a completely autologous reconstruction, insertion of an implant or expander implant may be necessary to achieve the desired breast size. Lipomodeling by Coleman fat transfer may be able to avoid implants and can also be used to augment the flap volume in case of volume loss postoperatively.[29,30] The effects of adjuvant radiotherapy on the completely autologous latissimus dorsi flap appear to be less detrimental than on the implant-based latissimus dorsi flap. Although radiotherapy may cause some reduction in the volume of the upper pole, the overall cosmetic outcome remains acceptable enough to advocate the autologous latissimus dorsi for immediate breast reconstruction.[11,31]

SHOULDER FUNCTION AFTER LATISSIMUS DORSI FLAP

Dorsal sequelae after autologous latissimus dorsi flaps are minimal and compare favourably with the morbidity caused by pedicled or free TRAM flaps.[32] The functional deficit after transfer of a latissimus dorsi muscle affects only very specific activities like rowing, cross-country skiing or mountain climbing but appears to have little affect on most other activities. There is a clinically significant reduction in function for up to 3 months but the recovery plateaus after 6 months and the long-term function is 'normal' in most patients. There is a potential for further impairment of a shoulder, which may have already been compromised by previous surgery.[33] Predictive patient-related, and therapeutic risk factors have been identified such as increasing body mass index and chest circumference, axillary surgery and pre-existing shoulder pathology.[34]

MAGNITUDE OF PROCEDURE

Latissimus dorsi breast reconstruction is a major operation but less involved than free tissue transfer. Approximately 3–4 hours operating time, a hospital stay of 7–10 days and a recovery time of 4–8 weeks are required.

INDICATIONS

The main indications for the latissimus dorsi flap include: (i) the reconstruction of larger and more pendulous breasts where an implant alone would not be sufficient for size; (ii) if the chest wall tissues are unsuitable for tissue expansion; and (iii) if there are additional tissue requirements after mastectomy (Fig. 4A,B). The latissimus dorsi is the workhorse flap for chest wall reconstruction or salvage surgery which may be required for advanced cancers and recurrent breast cancer after mastectomy or reconstruction (Fig. 5A–D).

Key point 5

- Salvage surgery with the latissimus dorsi flap may be required for complications of other reconstructions or for oncological reasons.

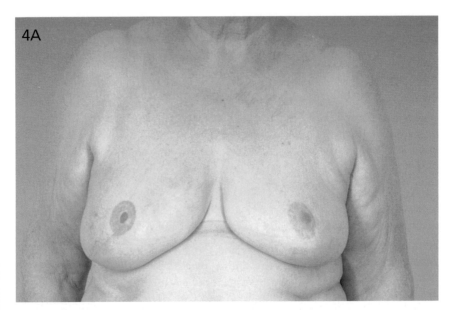

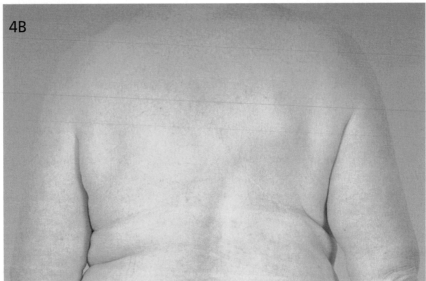

Fig. 4 (A) Immediate breast reconstruction with de-epithelialised autologous latissimus dorsi, buried completely under breast skin flaps, concomitant reduction of left breast. (B) Postoperative view of autologous latissimus dorsi donor site.

Further indications are bilateral breast reconstruction, contralateral reconstruction if abdominal tissues have already been used, congenital breast hypoplasia such as Poland's syndrome, replacement of implants with autologous tissue, partial breast reconstruction after conservation surgery or partial loss of an abdominal tissue flap (Figs 6A–E). The latissimus dorsi is ideal in patients with a moderate amount of body fat who have a full opposite breast with some ptosis and are not suitable for or do not want abdominal tissue breast reconstruction.[35–37]

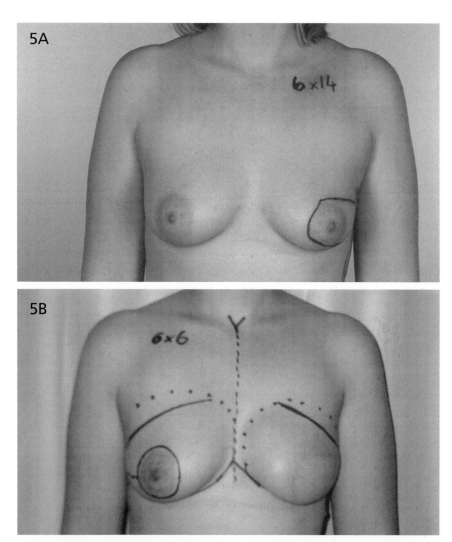

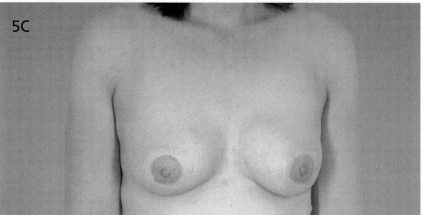

Fig. 5 Bilateral metachronous breast reconstruction with autologous latissimus dorsi in patient with right breast cancer and risk-reducing mastectomy on left breast after genetic testing. (A,B) Pre-operative views; (C,D) postoperative views of breast site and donor site.

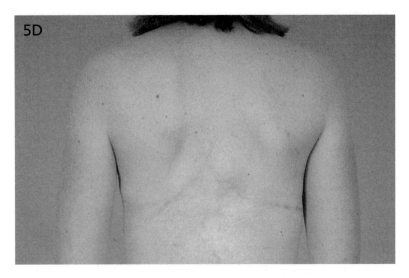

Fig. 5 *(continued)* (D) Postoperative view of the donor site.

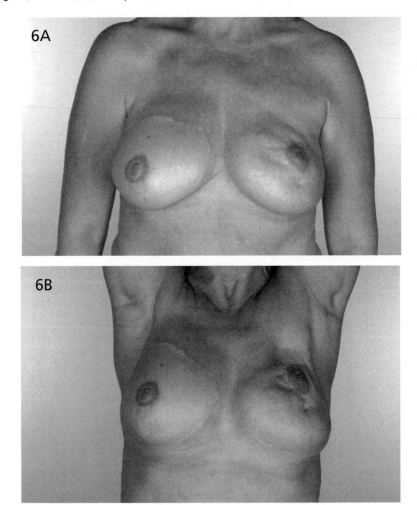

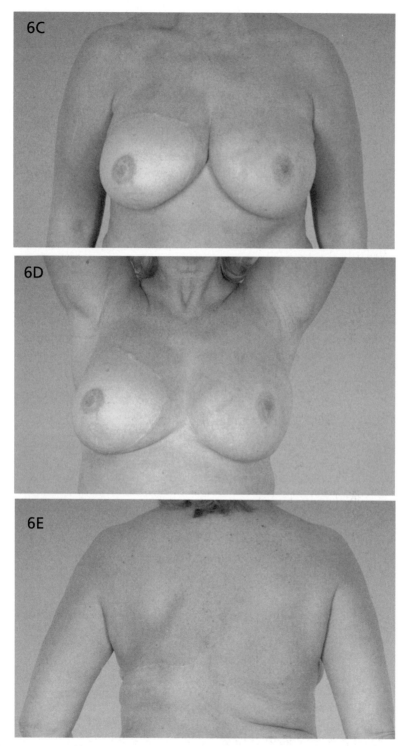

Fig. 6 Unacceptable appearance and synkinesia left breast after subcutaneous mastectomy and implant reconstruction. Right breast reconstructed with free DIEP flap. Replacement of implant with autologous latissimus dorsi flap. (A,B) Pre-operative views; (C–E) postoperative appearance of breast and donor site.

CONTRA-INDICATIONS

Contra-indications for latissimus dorsi breast reconstruction are previous surgery which may have compromised the vascular supply to the flap, absence of the latissimus dorsi muscle and serious patient co-morbidity.[1] This technique may not yield satisfactory results if there is a large defect involving breast skin and chest wall tissues. The latissimus dorsi flap with implant should not be used for immediate reconstruction if adjuvant radiotherapy is likely. The latissimus dorsi flap is unable to protect the underlying implant from the detrimental effects of radiotherapy; once the muscle has been irradiated, it can no longer be used for revision or replacement of the contracted implant with an autologous flap.[31]

Key point 6

- Implant-based latissimus dorsi reconstructions allow some control over breast size but have a high rate of symmetry and maintenance surgery. Further procedures may be required for complications and maintenance. Asymmetry may re-occur due to due to gravity and fluctuations in weight. The long-term outcome is directly related to the tolerance of breast implants and generally poor after radiotherapy.

SURGICAL TECHNIQUES

This technique is extremely versatile. The latissimus dorsi muscle can be transferred as muscle-only flap without a skin island to cover an implant or skin grafted if used for chest wall reconstruction. A myocutaneous flap can be used for chest wall resurfacing or may cover a breast implant or tissue expander for breast reconstruction. It is also possible to reconstruct a small-to-moderate size breast with an extended or autologous latissimus dorsi flap alone. A muscle sparing or perforator based technique, the so-called thoracodorsal artery perforator (T-DAP) flap, can be used for partial breast reconstruction or axillary resurfacing if preservation of muscle function is desirable.[13,18,28]

Key point 7 & 8

- The aesthetic results of autologous reconstruction are superior due to their versatility, their more natural appearance, consistency and durability. Autologous tissue can better withstand radiotherapy.

- The autologous latissimus dorsi flap is a safe and highly versatile technique which can provide a significant amount of soft tissue and has acceptable donor site morbidity.

SURGICAL TECHNIQUE OF THE AUTOLOGOUS LATISSIMUS DORSI FLAP

PRE-OPERATIVE PLANNING

The function of the latissimus dorsi muscle must be tested prior to surgery. If necessary, colour Doppler or MRI scanning can be used to establish the continuity of the thoracodorsal vessels. Pre-operative planning requires assessment of: size and shape of the opposite breast, the area of breast skin excision, the thickness and quality of the skin flaps in delayed breast reconstruction, the condition and function of the pectoralis major muscle, the position of the mastectomy scar and additional soft tissue requirements.

The amount and distribution of excess skin and soft tissue on the back are evaluated. A lean back can yield 300–400 cc, an average back 600–800 cc and a plump back 1200–1500 cc.

Prior to surgery, breast base, inframammary fold, anterior axillary fold, the take-off point of the breast, the limits of the latissimus dorsi muscle, areas of additional soft tissue harvest and the skin ellipse are marked. This ellipse should be centred over the fat roll on the back and positioned in the relaxed skin tension lines. The resulting scar should lie in the middle-to-lower bra strap area.

POSITIONING IN THE OPERATING THEATRE

The patient is positioned in a lateral decubitus position and secured with well-padded table attachments. The arm is supported at a 90° angle to allow access to the axilla. A combined approach in immediate reconstruction can save up to 1.5 hours' operating time but a separate incision may be required for the axillary clearance.

FLAP HARVEST

Infiltration with local anaesthetic and normal saline facilitates dissection. The skin island is incised and the skin flaps are raised at the level of Scarpa's fascia in order to protect the blood supply to the overlying skin flaps and ensure maximum soft tissue harvest with the flap. At the border of the previously marked flap, the dissection is carried down to latissimus dorsi muscle, the muscles overlying the scapula and the anterior border of the trapezius muscle. The adipofascial parascapular flap extension is lifted off the scapula and the upper edge of the latissimus dorsi muscle is exposed. The proximal portion of the muscle is dissected up to the tendineous insertion. The undersurface of the muscle can then be dissected. All intercostal perforators are divided and haemostasis is secured. The anterior border with the additional soft tissue anterior to the muscle is elevated last. Care has to be taken to avoid unintentional raising of the serratus anterior muscle and harvesting of slips of external oblique or serratus posterior muscles. As the latissimus dorsi is lifted off the serratus anterior, the neurovascular pedicle on the surface of the serratus and the serratus branch are identified and preserved. The posterior border of the latissimus dorsi muscle is detached from the teres muscles up to the tendineus insertion to allow the muscle to rotate to the anterior chest wall high up in the axilla. This avoids excess bulk on the lateral chest wall and augments the bulk of the anterior axillary fold at the same time. The anterior border of the muscle is freed, carefully avoiding damage to the thoracodorsal neurovascular bundle. The muscle is transferred through a high axillary tunnel. It is generally not necessary to divide the latissimus dorsi tendon or the serratus branch which can provide additional vascularity, particularly in delayed reconstruction when the main thoracodorsal vein may be encased by scar tissue. The thoracodorsal nerve is preserved in the autologous latissimus dorsi to maintain muscular bulk. Muscle twitching tends to decrease with time and is rarely a problem in completely autologous flaps. If used with an implant, synkinesia may result unless the nerve is divided. The donor site is closed in three layers with absorbable sutures after insertion of two drains. Quilting of the donor site can reduce the incidence of postoperative seroma.

FLAP INSET

The final flap inset is performed with the patient in a supine position. The upper part of the latissimus dorsi muscle is secured to the lateral border of the pectoralis major muscle and the flap is then rotated 180°. The parascapular adipofascial flap is folded under for extra projection in the lower pole. The edges of the flap are sutured into the borders of the mastectomy defect and the anterior axillary fold and the inframammary fold are recreated. Any excess skin island is de-epithelialised and projection can be adjusted with plication sutures. The size of the reconstructed breast should be about 25% larger than the opposite breast to allow for some postoperative atrophy.[35]

POSTOPERATIVE MANAGEMENT

A well-supported brassiere assists in the final moulding of the reconstructed breast. Physiotherapy should start on the first postoperative day with shoulder shrugging and exercises up to 90°. Rehabilitation of the scapular region follows after 4 weeks.[38]

COMPLICATIONS

Potential postoperative complications include wound failure, expander or implant failure and complications of breast implants. Flap-related wound complications are haematoma, infection, partial or total flap necrosis, breast skin necrosis and delayed healing. Donor site related complications include haematoma, seroma, wound infection, skin necrosis and wound dehiscence. Seroma formation is common after harvest of an extended and may require repeated aspiration. Several strategies have been suggested to reduce the incidence of postoperative seroma such as quilting sutures and the injection of topical steroids.[39]

Localised fat necrosis in autologous latissimus dorsi flaps has been reported in up to 14% of cases. Partial flap necrosis occurs in less than 5–7% of cases and total flap necrosis in less than 1% (Tables 1 and 2).[27,32,40]

SPECIFIC COMPLICATIONS

The incidence of implant failure and complications of breast implants are similar to implant-only reconstructions and include capsular contracture,

Table 1 Postoperative complications of latissimus dorsi flaps with and without implants

	Autologous latissimus dorsi	Latissimus dorsi with implant
Total flap loss	0–1%	0.6%
Partial flap loss	1–7%	3%
Fat necrosis	4–14%	3%
Breast skin necrosis	10%	19%
Wound infection	2%	5%

Table 2 Donor site complications of latissimus dorsi flaps.

	Autologous latissimus dorsi	Latissimus dorsi with implant
Seroma	3–80%	9%
Haematoma	3–6%	0.6%
Wound dehiscence	10–25%	16%

asymmetry, implant displacement and thinning of the overlying skin.[40] The commonest and least predictable complication of implant reconstruction is capsular contracture. Hardening of the scar tissue around the implant leads to firmness on palpation and distortion of the breast as well as discomfort and pain. Further surgical revision is often necessary. The risk of capsular contracture is significantly increased in the presence of infection and pre-operative or postoperative radiotherapy.[10,40] Although there is currently not enough information about the actual life-span of implants, maintenance surgery will be required in most cases. The average re-operation rate for an implant or tissue expander based breast reconstruction is 25% in the first 3 years and the rate of symmetry surgery to the opposite breast is about 60%.[41,42]

Key points for clinical practice

- Breast reconstruction plays a significant role in the woman's physical, emotional and psychological recovery from breast cancer.

- The ideal breast reconstruction is a soft, natural-feeling breast which maintains its characteristics over time as a natural ptosis or droop and a permanent and natural inframammary fold.

- Immediate breast reconstruction is safe, has no known oncological disadvantages, is most cost-effective and leads to the best cosmetic results due to maximum preservation of breast skin but exposes the reconstructions to the effects of radiotherapy.

- Delayed reconstruction involves a separate episode of hospitalisation, requires replacement of a larger amount of skin and potentially poor mastectomy flaps.

(continued on next page)

Key points for clinical practice *(continued)*

- Salvage surgery with the latissimus dorsi flap may be required for complications of other reconstructions or for oncological reasons.

- Implant-based latissimus dorsi reconstructions allow some control over breast size but have a high rate of symmetry and maintenance surgery. Further procedures may be required for complications and maintenance. Asymmetry may re-occur due to due to gravity and fluctuations in weight. The long-term outcome is directly related to the tolerance of breast implants and generally poor after radiotherapy.

- The aesthetic results of autologous reconstruction are superior due to their versatility, their more natural appearance, consistency and durability. Autologous tissue can better withstand radiotherapy.

- The autologous latissimus dorsi flap is a safe and highly versatile technique which can provide a significant amount of soft tissue and has acceptable donor site morbidity.

References

1. Weiler-Mithoff EM. Breast reconstruction: techniques, timing and patient selection. *Breast Cancer* 2001; **13**: 1–11.
2. British Association of Plastic Surgeons. *Oncoplastic Breast Surgery – A guide to good practice*. British Association of Plastic Surgeons, Educational programme: Course 3: Breast, 31 March – 1 April 2006; 11–23.
3. Kroll SS, Ames F, Singletary SE, Schusterman MA. The oncologic risks of skin preservation at mastectomy when combined with immediate reconstruction of the breast. *Surg Gynecol Obstet* 1991; **172**: 17–20.
4. Bensimon RH, Bergmeyer JM. Improved aesthetics in breast reconstruction: modified mastectomy incision and immediate autologous tissue reconstruction. *Ann Plast Surg* 1995; **34**: 229–233.
5. Brown IM, Wilson CR, Weiler-Mithoff EM, George WD, Doughty JC. Immediate breast reconstruction does not lead to a delay in the delivery of adjuvant chemotherapy. *Eur J Surg Oncol* 2004; **30**: 624–627.
6. Malata CM, McIntosh SA, Prurushotham AD. Immediate breast reconstruction after mastectomy for cancer. *Br J Surg* 2000; **87**: 1455–1472.
7. Rosenquist S, Sandelin K, Wickmann M. Patients' psychological and cosmetic experience after immediate breast reconstruction. *Eur J Surg Oncol* 1996; **22**: 262–266.
8. Noone RB, Frazier TG, Noone GC, Blanhet NP, Murphy JB, Rose D. Recurrence of breast carcinoma following immediate reconstruction: a 13-year review. *Plast Reconstr Surg* 1994; **93**: 90–106.
9. Godfrey PM, Godfrey NV, Romita MC. Immediate autogenous breast reconstruction in clinically advanced disease. *Plast Reconstr Surg* 1995; **95**: 1039–1044.
10. Hussien M, Salah B, Malyon A, Weiler-Mithoff EM. Impact of adjuvant radiotherapy on the choice of immediate breast reconstruction. *Eur J Cancer* 2000; **36 (Suppl. 5)**: 58.
11. Brown IM, Hogg FJ, McKown DJ, Weiler-Mithoff EM, Scott JR. Long term aesthetic outcome of immediate breast reconstruction with the autologous latissimus dorsi flap with or without adjuvant radiotherapy. Dublin: BAPS Summer Meeting, 2004.
12. Bostwick III J. *Plastic and Reconstructive Breast Surgery*. St Louis, MO: Quality Medical Publishing, 1990.

13. Cormack GC, Lamberty GH. *The Arterial Anatomy of Skin Flaps*, 2nd edn. Edinburgh: Churchill Livingstone, 1994.

14. Maxwell GP. Iginio Tansini and the origin of the latissimus dorsi musculocutaneous flap. *Plast Reconstr Surg* 1980; **65**: 686–692.

15. Olivari N. The latissimus flap. *Br J Plast Surg* 1976; **29**: 126–128.

16. Muehlbauer W, Olbrisch RR. The latissimus dorsi myo-cutaneous flap for breast reconstruction. *Chir Plast* 1977; **4**: 27–34.

17. McCraw JB, Papp CTh. Latissimus dorsi myocutaneous flap. In: Hartrampf CR. (ed) *Breast Reconstruction with Living Tissue*. Norfolk, VA: Hampton Press, 1991; 211–248.

18. Schneider WJ, Hill HJ, Brown RG. Latissimus dorsi myo-cutaneous flap for breast reconstruction. *Br J Plast Surg* 1977; **30**: 281-288.

19. Bostwick III J, Vasconez LO, Jurkiewicz MJ. Breast reconstruction after a radical mastectomy. *Plast Reconstr Surg* 1978; **61**: 682–693.

20. Boehme PE. Mammaconstruction mit dem versenkten Latissimus dorsi Insellappen. In: Bohment H. (ed) *Brustkrebs und Brustkrebsrekonstruktion*. Stuttgart; Georg Thieme, 1982.

21. Papp C, Zanon E, McCraw JB. Breast volume replacement using the de-epithelialized latissimus dorsi myo-cutaneous flap. *Eur J Plast Surg* 1988; **11**: 120.

22. Hokin JA. Mastectomy reconstruction without a prosthetic implant. *Plast Reconstr Surg* 1983; **72**: 810.

23. Marshall DR, Anstee EJ, Stapleton MJ. Soft tissue reconstruction of the breast using an extended composite latissimus dorsi myo-cutaneous flap. *Br J Plast Surg* 1984; **37**: 361.

24. McCraw JB, Papp CT. Latissimus dorsi myo-cutaneous flap: 'Fleur de Lys' reconstruction. In Hartrampf CR. (ed) *Breast Reconstruction with Living Tissue*. Norfolk, VA: Hampton Press, 1991; 211.

25. Barnet GR, Gianoutsos MP. The latissimus dorsi added fat flap for natural tissue breast reconstruction: report of 15 cases. *Plast Reconstr Surg* 1996; **97**: 63–70.

26. Germann G, Steinau HU. Breast reconstruction with the extended latissimus dorsi flap. *Plast Reconstr Surg* 1996; **97**: 519.

27. Delay E, Gounot N, Bouillot A, Zlatoff P. Autologous latissimus breast reconstruction: a 3 year clinical experience with 100 patients. *Plast Reconstr Surg* 1998; **102**: 1461–1478.

28. Chang DW, Youssef A, Cha Sumi, Reece GP. Autologous breast reconstruction with the extended latissimus dorsi flap. *Plast Reconstr Surg* 2002; **110**: 751.

29. Fatah MFT. Extended latissimus dorsi flap in breast reconstruction. In: Culbertson JH, Jones G. (eds) *Operative Techniques in Plastic and Reconstructive Surgery*. New York: WB Saunders 1999; 38–49.

30. Delay E. Lipomodelling of the reconstructed breast. In: Spear SL. (ed) *Surgery of the Breast: Principles and Art*, 2nd edn. Philadelphia, PA: Lippincott-Raven, 2006; 930.

31. Scott JR, Malyon A, Hussien M, Weiler-Mithoff EM. Immediate breast reconstruction – the effect of adjuvant radiotherapy on latissimus dorsi flap reconstructions with and without implants. Stirling: BAPS Summer Meeting, 2001.

32. Clough KB, Louis-Sylvestre C, Fitoussi A, Couturaud B, Nos C. Donor site sequelae after autologous breast reconstruction with an extended latissimus dorsi flap. *Plast Reconstr Surg* 2002; **109**: 1904–1911.

33. Russell RC, Pribaz J, Zook EG, Leighton WD, Eriksson E, Smith CJ. Functional evaluation of latissimus dorsi donor site. *Plast Reconstr Surg* 1986; **78**: 336–344.

34. Button J, Hart AM, Tagizadeh R, Weiler-Mithoff EM, Scott JR. Shoulder function after autologous latissimus dorsi breast reconstruction: a prospective two-year observational study with comparison of quilting and non-quilting techniques. London: BAPS Winter Meeting, 2005.

35. Weiler-Mithoff EM. Breast reconstruction. In: Dixon M. (ed) *A Companion to Specialist Surgical Practice, Breast Surgery*, 3rd edn. Amsterdam: Elsevier, 2005; 117–132.

36. Baildam AD. Oncoplastic surgery of the breast. *Br J Surg* 2002; **89**: 532.

37. Audretsch WP. Reconstruction of the partial mastectomy defect: classification and method. In: Spear SL. (ed) *Surgery of the Breast: Principles and Art*. Philadelphia, PA: Lippincot-Raven, 1998; 155–169.

38. Futter C. Appendix: Physiotherapy following breast reconstruction. In: *Oncoplastic Breast Surgery – A guide to good practice*. British Association of Plastic Surgeons, Educational programme: Course 3: Breast, 31 March – 1 April 2006; 11–23, 77–84.

39. Taghizadeh R, Hart A, Shoaib T, Weiler-Mithoff EM. Seroma reduction in extended latissimus dorsi flap donor sites by injection of Triamcinolone – results of a randomised controlled trial. *J Plast Reconstr Aesth Surg* 2006; In press.

40. Roy MK, Shrotia S, Holcombe C, Webster DJT, Hughes LE, Mansel RE. Complications of latissimus dorsi myocutaneous flap breast reconstruction. *Eur J Surg Oncol* 1998; **24**: 162–165.

41. Clough KB, O'Donoghue JM, Fitoussi AD, Nos C, Falcou M-C. Prospective evaluation of late cosmetic results following breast reconstruction: implant reconstruction. *Plast Reconstr Surg* 2001: **107**: 1702–1709.

42. Gabriel SE, Woods JE, O'Fallon WM, Beard CM, Kurland LT, Melton 3rd LJ. Complications leading to surgery after breast implantation. *N Engl J Med* 1997; **336**: 677–682.

Thomas Armstrong James A. Pain

8

Acute gallbladder disease

This chapter focuses on contemporary management of the acute gallbladder and does not cover choledocholithiasis and its complications. Where possible, 'best practice' is considered in the context (and constraints) of British practice.

The overall prevalence of gallstones in adults is about 10% of whom approximately 1–2% per annum becomes symptomatic.[1,2] Two-thirds have been found to remain asymptomatic in long-term studies.[2] Emergency admission with acute gallbladder disease is common, accounting for at least 5% of acute surgical admissions in the UK.[3] Traditionally, patients have been managed conservatively in the emergency setting, with interval surgery planned on an elective basis. However, this strategy has been challenged for two reasons.

1. There is a high rate of morbidity amongst patients during this interval. Some 11–24% of patients with gallstone-related disease are admitted whilst waiting for laparoscopic cholecystectomy.[4,5] Moreover, those who present as an emergency (the majority with acute cholecystitis) have an even higher re-admission rate (29–40%) whilst waiting for surgery.[4,6] This is not only adverse for the patient but it has been estimated that each such admission has an associated cost of £1000 (admission for elective laparoscopic cholecystectomy costs £1700).[5]

2. Laparoscopic surgery has evolved in experience, techniques and equipment. Laparoscopic cholecystectomy is now regarded as safe during

Thomas Armstrong PhD MRCSEd (for correspondence)
Specialist Registrar, Department of General Surgery, Poole Hospital, Longfleet Road, Poole, Dorset BH15 2JB, UK
E-mail: armstrongthomas@talk21.com

James A. Pain MS FRCS
Consultant Surgeon, Department of General Surgery, Poole Hospital, Longfleet Road, Poole, Dorset BH15 2JB, UK

the index admission and many experts in this field would agree that this represents the optimum timing for surgery.[7]

Although there is plenty of evidence that early laparoscopic cholecystectomy is beneficial, it is important that it is used in the correct circumstances for the correct pathology. Consequently, an accurate diagnosis and a good understanding of the pathology underlying acute gallbladder diseases are required. The pathology can be broadly divided into acute calculous and acalculous cholecystitis, biliary colic and other gallbladder abnormalities (*e.g.* sludge and polyps). These are discussed separately but clearly, in practice, there will be overlap between conditions.

Key point 1

- Laparoscopic cholecystectomy is a safe treatment for acute cholecystitis and biliary colic during index admission, reducing hospital stay and preventing re-admission.

ACUTE CALCULOUS CHOLECYSTITIS

DIAGNOSIS

Acute cholecystitis occurs in up to 10% of patients with gallstones and is more likely if gallstones have previously been symptomatic.[2] Acute cholecystitis should be differentiated from biliary colic by the presence of constant pain in the right upper quadrant (> 12 hours), tenderness in right upper quadrant (usually with a positive Murphy's sign and sometimes a palpable mass) and a systemic inflammatory response (with raised inflammatory markers).[8] In the presence of these features, diagnosis is usually confirmed by ultrasonography.[9] The diagnostic characteristics being a thick-walled (> 3 mm), often distended, gall bladder containing gallstones (one of which may be impacted in Hartmann's pouch) and pericholecystic fluid collections may be present.[9] Eliciting Murphy's sign with the ultrasound probe is said to be useful. Ultrasound is operator-dependent and may have a sensitivity of only 50–60% in diagnosing acute cholecystitis.[10,11] If ultrasonography is not consistent with the clinical diagnosis, either the scan can be repeated or a different imaging modality used. Biliary cholescintigraphy (using hydroxyiminodiacetic acid [HIDA]) increases sensitivity to 80–90% but is rarely used in the UK.[10,11] Computed tomography (CT) is increasingly recognised as helpful, where ultrasound findings are equivocal and it is often useful in this scenario, with the benefit of identifying other pathology such as appendicitis, pancreatitis and perforated peptic ulcers.[12]

Deranged liver function tests or a dilated common bile duct should alert to the possibility of choledocholithiasis, which is reported to occur in up to 23% of patients with acute cholecystitis.[13] Magnetic resonance cholangio-pancreatography (MRCP) identifies bile duct stones with a high degree of sensitivity (81–100%) and specificity (92–100%); in conjunction with ultrasound, it can also exclude Mirizzi syndrome.[14] The presence of bile duct stone will determine whether a patient requires peri-operative endoscopic duct clearance (ERCP) or planned duct clearance during surgery.

MANAGEMENT

Medical

Most patients will respond to conservative treatment – analgesia, intravenous fluids, gastrointestinal rest and appropriate antibiotic therapy. This should be instituted on diagnosis regardless of whether surgery is planned. Bacterial infection can be identified in 80% of patients with cholecystitis.[15] It is caused by a variety of organisms (Table 1) and polymicrobial infection can be expected in half, with anaerobic infections occurring in about 10%. Antimicrobial therapy should be directed toward these organisms and quinolones (*e.g.* ciprofloxacin), cephalosporins (*e.g.* cefuroxime), penicillins (*e.g.* co-amoxiclavulanic acid) have the appropriate spectrum of activity. Diabetics are particularly prone to gangrenous and emphysematous cholecystitis. They should be closely monitored and given anaerobic cover (*e.g.* metronidazole). Principally for logistical reasons, 90% of British surgeons would perform an interval cholecystectomy at 6–12 weeks after resolution of the acute episode.[16] In this interval, 15–18% of patients will still require urgent surgery (*i.e.* those who fail to settle or develop serious complications such as gallbladder necrosis or perforation).[4,6] However, there is much good evidence that all patients should have urgent surgery.

Surgical

It has been established that urgent, open cholecystectomy for acute cholecystitis is safe, can reduce hospital stay and lead to a more rapid recovery.[16] This question has been re-examined since the advent of laparoscopic surgery because, in the pioneering days, acute cholecystitis was considered a contra-indication. There is plenty of data supporting the role of laparoscopic cholecystectomy during index admission for acute cholecystitis and this is analysed in depth in excellent reviews by Bhattacharya, Kitano, Liu and the meta-analysis by Papi and Lau.[17–21] The following summarises data presented in these reviews and articles cited therein.

Definition: Urgent cholecystectomy is defined as within 72–96 hours, delayed after 72–96 hours but during index admission and interval at 6–12 weeks. There is some cross-over between urgent and delayed as there is no consensus in definition in the literature.

Table 1 Bacteria isolated from bile in acute cholecystitis[15]

Common	*Escherichia coli*
	Enterococcus spp.
	Klebsiella pneumoniae
Others	*Morganell morganii*
	Pseudomonas aeruginosa
	Citrobacter freundii
	Enterobacter spp.
	Streptococcus Group D
	Salmonella spp.
	Bacteroides fragilis
	Clostridium perfringens

Urgent versus interval laparoscopic cholecystectomy

Four randomised trials (total 398 patients) have compared urgent versus interval laparoscopic cholecystectomy for acute calculous cholecystitis. These are summarised in Table 2 and show that urgent laparoscopic surgery for acute cholecystitis takes the same length of time, with similar complication rates as interval surgery but significantly reduces hospital stay. Interestingly, a recent, small but randomised trial of urgent laparoscopic versus open cholecystectomy showed little difference in clinically relevant postoperative outcome.[22]

Table 2 Summary of four randomised controlled trials (*n* = 398 patients) comparing urgent versus interval laparoscopic cholecystectomy[17]

	Operating time (min)	Conversion rate (%)	Complication rate (%)	Median hospital stay (days)
Urgent group	98–123	11–31	6–20	4–7.6
Interval group	90–106	23–29	8–29	8–11.6
Significant	No	No	No	Yes

Urgent versus delayed laparoscopic cholecystectomy

In the first 72–96 hours that symptoms are present, the inflammatory changes around the gallbladder tend to be oedematous, with tissue planes preserved, thus facilitating removal of the gallbladder. After this time frame, the acute inflammatory reaction progresses and matures with fibrotic changes predominating, obliterating tissue planes.[8] In practice, this is somewhat arbitrary, especially when the presentation is acute on chronic. In eight studies comparing urgent (*i.e.* within 72–96 hours of admission) versus delayed (beyond 72–96 hours but during the index admission), conversion rates of 0–27% increased to 17–60% (a significant increase in most studies). Furthermore, average operating time increased in the order of 10–30 min in those studies which included these data (significantly so in three). Complication rates quoted in 6 of 8 studies varied between 12–30% and there was no difference between groups. The median total hospital stay significantly increased in all studies from a median of 2.1–8.3 days in the urgent group to 7.1–22.3 days in the delayed group. Other authors have found that the timing of surgery makes little difference and it is the degree of inflammation that is important.[23] Data comparing urgent and delayed groups must be interpreted carefully, because only one of the eight studies was truly randomised and this showed minimal differences (although the groups were small). Inevitably, the delayed group will spend longer in hospital because surgery was delayed. However, if surgery is performed within 72–96 hours, it is likely to be technically easier, with fewer conversions and allow patients to get home sooner without the risk of re-admission.

The timing of surgery is not the only predictor for open conversion; male sex, advancing age, obesity, gall bladder wall thickening and the presence of a palpable gallbladder and complicated cholecystitis are also important.[19]

Surgical technique

It is widely recognised amongst those practising laparoscopic surgery that complications are fewer in experienced hands. Surgeons should be competent to undertake elective laparoscopic cholecystectomy prior to tackling acute cholecystitis because this surgery is technically more challenging. Several technical modifications are suggested when performing laparoscopic surgery for acute cholecystitis. It may be useful to use a 30° laparoscope, additional ports and retractors. Grasping and retracting the acutely inflamed gallbladder can be facilitated by decompressing the gallbladder or inserting a suture and retracting it via the abdominal wall. Blunt dissection is useful, including hydrostatic dissection. An endoloop rather than clips may be used to ligate the cystic duct. At completion of the procedure, the gallbladder can be removed in a bag and the use of a sub-hepatic drain considered.[19,24] Conversion to an open operation is required if it is not possible to satisfactorily demonstrate the anatomy.

Key point 2 & 3

- Laparoscopic cholecystectomy may be technically easier within 72–96 hours of acute cholecystitis developing.

- Laparoscopic cholecystectomy in the acute setting should be carried out by an experienced surgeon.

Intra-operative cholangiography

Intra-operative cholangiography (IOC) may help define anatomy but, as in the elective setting, there is no consensus if this should be selective or routine. It may be technically more difficult to perform IOC in acute cholecystitis. The rate of unexpected choledocholithiasis is reported to be similar to that observed in all patients undergoing elective cholecystectomy (5%); on this basis, normal local practice should be adopted.[17] An alternative to IOC is intra-operative ultrasound but this will depend on availability and local expertise. Laparoscopic bile duct clearance is feasible during surgery for acute cholecystitis but it remains a matter of debate whether this is preferable to peri-operative duct clearance with ERCP.[25] Inevitably, local expertise, enthusiasm and resource will determine how choledocholithiasis is managed.

Complications of surgery

The most common serious complication following cholecystectomy is damage to the bile ducts, which is associated with a 1.5–6% mortality. There is an 8–20% risk of major morbidity associated with biliary-enteric reconstruction, principally due to anastomotic strictures causing acute and chronic cholangitis and, less commonly, secondary biliary cirrhosis.[26–29] In the review by Bhattacharya and Ammori,[17] the observed rate of bile duct injury during laparoscopic cholecystectomy in acute cholecystitis was 0.7% in 994 patients compared to 0.5% in studies of interval cholecystectomy. In other large studies, the overall incidence of bile duct injury for all patients is approximately 0.3–0.5%, typified by a recent Italian study in which the rate of bile duct injury was 0.42% amongst 56,591 patients.[30] This study identified a significantly increased risk of bile duct injury in patients with previous cholecystitis (0.56%) compared with simple biliary colic (0.32%). Biliary leaks appear to occur following about 2.5% of urgent and interval laparoscopic cholecystectomy and cause transient morbidity only.[17] Hence, there is likely to be a small increase in bile duct damage associated with urgent laparoscopic surgery for acute cholecystitis but rates of minor complications are similar to interval surgery.

Percutaneous cholecystostomy

In patients who are considered unfit for cholecystectomy, either secondary to severe sepsis or co-morbidity, percutaneous cholecystostomy provides an alternative to laparoscopic cholecystectomy. Many studies of the use of percutaneous cholecystectomy include data from patients who have acalculous cholecystitis and it is difficult to ascertain the proportion of patients with calculous cholecystitis who subsequently have laparoscopic cholecystectomy but it appears to be approximately 50%. Percutaneous cholecystectomy may allow resolution of sepsis and permit delayed or interval surgery where co-morbidity needs optimisation.[31] Percutaneous cholecystectomy is performed radiologically using a modified Seldinger technique under ultrasound or CT guidance.[32] A 'pigtail'-type catheter is inserted via transperitoneal or, ideally, the transhepatic route.[31,32] Potential complications include bleeding, bile leak, bowel perforation, pneumothorax and tube blockage/displacement.[32] A cholecystogram may not be appropriate at the time of initial insertion of a percutaneous cholecystostomy if sepsis is present but can be performed after 2–3 days or when clinical condition allows. A cholecystogram will help rule out gallbladder carcinoma and contrast may pass into the biliary tree (especially if bile had been draining from the tube) allowing identification of bile duct stones. A mature track will form after 2 weeks and the tube should be left in for at least this period.

Some authors have used percutaneous cholecystostomy as a precursor to early laparoscopic cholecystectomy.[15] In a large, but non-randomised, trial ($n = 145$), all patients admitted with an empyaema underwent percutaneous cholecystectomy, with immediate improvement in 93% of patients. Subsequently, 80% of patients underwent laparoscopic cholecystectomy after a mean of 4 days (range, 2–22 days). There was a 27% conversion rate, 17% complication rate, 2.6% mortality rate and bile duct injuries in 1.4% of patients.[15] Studies of interval laparoscopic cholecystectomy after percutaneous cholecystectomy have shown similar rates of complication and conversion.[31] Therefore, percutaneous cholecystectomy has a role in managing calculous cholecystitis.

Key point 4 & 5

- Percutaneous cholecystostomy is a useful intervention for patients with acute cholecystitis who are not fit for laparoscopic cholecystectomy (e.g. severe sepsis or co-morbidity).

- Percutaneous cholecystostomy is the treatment of choice for acalculous cholecystitis.

Conclusions

There is little doubt that laparoscopic cholecystectomy during the index admission now has an established role in treating acute gallbladder disease and is likely to become the gold standard in treatment. However, there remain significant logistical problems in achieving this in most British surgical units. There are often delays in getting the appropriate imaging in order to operate within the first 72–96 hours. Emergency ('CEPOD') lists are often overstretched, with several specialties competing for theatre time. Furthermore, surgical staff with adequate experience are not always available. It is important that the limited available resource for performing surgery in the NHS is fully utilised; therefore, planned, interval surgery will necessarily continue in many units.

In larger surgical units, a specialist-led service may overcome some of these problems and care pathways can improve and regulate such services.[24,33] With the planned changes in training and staffing of surgical units combined with the reduction in number of 'acute' hospitals, it may become possible to offer this service throughout the NHS.

Key point 6

- Logistical problems currently prevent the provision of urgent laparoscopic cholecystectomy in many British surgical units.

BILIARY COLIC

Biliary colic can be differentiated from acute cholecystitis by the presence of shorter, self-limiting attacks of pain, which are not associated with signs of inflammation. The gallbladder is typically 'thin walled' on ultrasonography (although there is clearly some overlap between biliary colic, acute and chronic cholecystitis). There is a trend towards performing laparoscopic cholecystectomy in patients who present acutely with biliary colic on the index admission.[23,34,35] This prevents the potentially high re-admission rate of these patients.[35] The timing of surgery in patients without inflammation is less important.

ACUTE ACALCULOUS CHOLECYSTITIS

Compared to the diagnosis of acute cholecystitis, acalculous cholecystitis presents more of a diagnostic challenge. It is typically seen in patients who are critically ill or who have undergone major trauma or surgery but is also seen in a variety of medical illnesses (Table 3). The mortality rate associated with the condition is about 30%.[36] In trauma patients (multiple injuries and burns), 90% of those who develop cholecystitis have acalculous cholecystitis, in contrast to the post-surgical group (often cardiac/vascular surgery) of whom half have calculous cholecystitis. The vast majority of patients (up to 80%) are male. More than half of all cases of cholecystitis in children are acalculous.[36]

The proposed pathogenesis of acalculous cholecystitis is believed to be related to bile stasis and gallbladder ischaemia.[36] Bile stasis occurs partly as a result of volume depletion and gastrointestinal hypomotility, which may be exacerbated by opiate-induced sphincter of Oddi dysfunction. Furthermore, positive pressure ventilation may increase hepatic venous pressure thus decreasing portal perfusion pressure and promoting bile stasis. Gallbladder hypoperfusion can be a direct consequence of the precipitating illness (*e.g.* vasculitis, atherosclerosis) or as a result of hypovolaemia and concomitant use of vasopressors. It is clear why it is seen in critically ill patients but not so clear why it should particularly affect men.

Table 3 Conditions associated with acalculous cholecystitis[36]

Trauma	
Surgery	Vascular
	Cardiac
Cardiovascular	Congestive cardiac failure
	Atherosclerosis
Endocrine	Diabetes mellitus
Immunological	Systemic lupus erythematosis
	Polyarteritis nodosa
Infection	*Candida* spp.
	Salmonella spp.
	Cholera
	Tuberculosis
	Malaria
	Brucellosis
	Aschariasis
	Human immunodeficiency virus

The diagnostic challenge lies in the type of patient that typically develops acalculous cholecystitis. They are often critically ill and obtunded, with several potential sources of sepsis already present and derangement of liver biochemistry possibly attributable to other aspects of their illness or treatment.[36] When suspected, the diagnosis can be confirmed using ultrasound. A gallbladder wall thickness of 3.5 mm, without gallstones allows diagnosis with 98.5% specificity and 80% sensitivity. CT scanning has been shown to be equally good in diagnosing acalculous cholecystitis. False-positives may occur with gallbladder sludge or iso-echoic calculi.[37]

Accurate diagnosis is vital because, in the case of true acalculous cholecystitis, a percutaneous cholecystostomy may be the only treatment required. Subsequent interval cholecystectomy is rarely required.[36]

SLUDGE AND POLYPS

Gallbladder sludge and polyps are occasionally noted on ultrasound in those patients who suffer acute right upper quadrant pain. Biliary sludge is essentially microlithiasis and is arbitrarily differentiated from calculi when particles are < 2 mm in diameter. These sediments are comprised of cholesterol microcrystals and pigment material and are assumed to be a precursor of gallstone formation. Microlithiasis is predisposed by bile stasis.[38] Biliary sludge is found in up to 30% of pregnant women (usually resolves after cessation of pregnancy), 50% of patients treated with TPN, 67% of patients following bone marrow/solid organ transplant, 25% of patients following obesity surgery and up to 40% after treatment with certain drugs (*e.g.*

ceftriaxone and octreotide). In common with calculous disease, it is estimated that 10% of patients with biliary sludge will become symptomatic but in 50% sludge will disappear.[39] Therefore, in the acute setting, treatment should be symptomatic and expectant, particularly where there is a correctable cause with surgery reserved for those with persistent symptoms or complications (*e.g.* pancreatitis).[38,39]

The majority of gallbladder polyps are simply misdiagnosed gallstones.[40] In those who have lesions genuinely originating from the gallbladder wall, two-thirds will be cholesterol polyps (accumulations of fat-filled macrophages) and the remainder will be inflammatory, hyperplastic or neoplastic polyps. It is, therefore, recommended that 'polyps' demonstrated in the presence of symptoms undergo interval cholecystectomy. In the absence of symptoms, any patients with solitary polyps greater than 10 mm in diameter should undergo cholecystectomy because of the higher incidence of neoplastic transformation.[40]

Key points for clinical practice

- Laparoscopic cholecystectomy is a safe treatment for acute cholecystitis and biliary colic during index admission, reducing hospital stay and preventing re-admission.

- Laparoscopic cholecystectomy may be technically easier within 72–96 hours of acute cholecystitis developing.

- Laparoscopic cholecystectomy in the acute setting should be carried out by an experienced surgeon.

- Percutaneous cholecystostomy is a useful intervention for patients with acute cholecystitis who are not fit for laparoscopic cholecystectomy (*e.g.* severe sepsis or co-morbidity).

- Percutaneous cholecystostomy is the treatment of choice for acalculous cholecystitis.

- Logistical problems currently prevent the provision of urgent laparoscopic cholecystectomy in many British surgical units..

References

1. Bates T, Harrison M, Lowe D, Lawson C, Padley N. Longitudinal study of gall stone prevalence at necropsy. *Gut* 1992; **33**: 103–107.
2. Friedman GD. Natural history of asymptomatic and symptomatic gallstones. *Am J Surg* 1993; **165**: 399–404.
3. Irvin TT. Abdominal pain: a surgical audit of 1190 emergency admissions. *Br J Surg* 1989; **76**: 1121–1125.
4. Cheruvu CV, Eyre-Brook IA. Consequences of prolonged wait before gallbladder surgery. *Ann R Coll Surg Engl* 2002; **84**: 20–22.
5. Somasekar K, Shankar PJ, Foster ME, Lewis MH. Costs of waiting for gall bladder surgery. *Postgrad Med J* 2002; **78**: 668–669.
6. Cameron IC, Chadwick C, Phillips J, Johnson AG. Acute cholecystitis – room for improvement? *Ann R Coll Surg Engl* 2002; **84**: 10–13.
7. Gouma DJ. Conversion from laparoscopic to open cholecystectomy. *Br J Surg* 2006; **93**: 905–906.

8. Indar AA, Beckingham IJ. Acute cholecystitis. *BMJ* 2002; **325**: 639–643.

9. Rubens DJ. Hepatobiliary imaging and its pitfalls. *Radiol Clin North Am* 2004; **42**: 257–278.

10. Kalimi R, Gecelter GR, Caplin D *et al*. Diagnosis of acute cholecystitis: sensitivity of sonography, cholescintigraphy, and combined sonography-cholescintigraphy. *J Am Coll Surg* 2001; **193**: 609–613.

11. Alobaidi M, Gupta R, Jafri SZ, Fink-Bennet DM. Current trends in imaging evaluation of acute cholecystitis. *Emerg Radiol* 2004; **10**: 256–258.

12. Bennett GL, Balthazar EJ. Ultrasound and CT evaluation of emergent gallbladder pathology. *Radiol Clin North Am* 2003; **41**: 1203–1216.

13. Hsieh CH. Early minilaparoscopic cholecystectomy in patients with acute cholecystitis. *Am J Surg* 2003; **185**: 344–348.

14. Freitas ML, Bell RL, Duffy AJ. Choledocholithiasis: evolving standards for diagnosis and management. *World J Gastroenterol* 2006; **12**: 3162–3167.

15. Tseng LJ, Tsai CC, Mo LR *et al*. Palliative percutaneous transhepatic gallbladder drainage of gallbladder empyema before laparoscopic cholecystectomy. *Hepatogastroenterology* 2000; **47**: 932–936.

16. Cameron IC, Chadwick C, Phillips J, Johnson AG. Management of acute cholecystitis in UK hospitals: time for a change. *Postgrad Med J* 2004; **80**: 292–294.

17. Bhattacharya D, Ammori BJ. Contemporary minimally invasive approaches to the management of acute cholecystitis: a review and appraisal. *Surg Laparosc Endosc Percutan Tech* 2005; **15**: 1–8.

18. Kitano S, Matsumoto T, Aramaki M, Kawano K. Laparoscopic cholecystectomy for acute cholecystitis. *J Hepatobiliary Pancreat Surg* 2002; **9**: 534–537.

19. Liu TH, Consorti ET, Mercer DW. Laparoscopic cholecystectomy for acute cholecystitis: technical considerations and outcome. *Semin Laparosc Surg* 2002; **9**: 24–31.

20. Papi C, Catarci M, D'Ambrosio L *et al*. Timing of cholecystectomy for acute calculous cholecystitis: a meta-analysis. *Am J Gastroenterol* 2004; **99**: 147–155.

21. Lau H, Lo CY, Patil NG, Yuen WK. Early versus delayed-interval laparoscopic cholecystectomy for acute cholecystitis: a meta-analysis. *Surg Endosc* 2006; **20**: 82–87.

22. Johansson M, Thune A, Nelvin L, Stiernstam M, Westman B, Lundell L. Randomized clinical trial of open versus laparoscopic cholecystectomy in the treatment of acute cholecystitis. *Br J Surg* 2005; **92**: 44–49.

23. Knight JS, Mercer SJ, Somers SS, Walters AM, Sadek SA, Toh SK. Timing of urgent laparoscopic cholecystectomy does not influence conversion rate. *Br J Surg* 2004; **91**: 601–604.

24. Mercer SJ, Knight JS, Toh SK, Walters AM, Sadek SA, Somers SS. Implementation of a specialist-led service for the management of acute gallstone disease. *Br J Surg* 2004; **91**: 504–508.

25. Decker G, Borie F, Millat B *et al*. One hundred laparoscopic choledochotomies with primary closure of the common bile duct. *Surg Endosc* 2003; **17**: 12–18.

26. Moraca RJ, Lee FT, Ryan Jr JA, Traverso LW. Long-term biliary function after reconstruction of major bile duct injuries with hepaticoduodenostomy or hepaticojejunostomy. *Arch Surg* 2002; **137**: 889–893.

27. Frilling A, Li J, Weber F *et al*. Major bile duct injuries after laparoscopic cholecystectomy: a tertiary center experience. *J Gastrointest Surg* 2004; **8**: 679–685.

28. Sicklick JK, Camp MS, Lillemoe KD *et al*. Surgical management of bile duct injuries sustained during laparoscopic cholecystectomy: perioperative results in 200 patients. *Ann Surg* 2005; **241**: 786–792.

29. Schmidt SC, Langrehr JM, Hintze RE, Neuhaus P. Long-term results and risk factors influencing outcome of major bile duct injuries following cholecystectomy. *Br J Surg* 2005; **92**: 76–82.

30. Nuzzo G, Giuliante F, Giovannini I *et al*. Bile duct injury during laparoscopic cholecystectomy: results of an Italian national survey on 56 591 cholecystectomies. *Arch Surg* 2005; **140**: 986–992.

31. Johnson AB, Fink AS. Alternative methods for management of the complicated gallbladder. *Semin Laparosc Surg* 1998; **5**: 115–120.

32. Akhan O, Akinci D, Ozmen MN. Percutaneous cholecystostomy. *Eur J Radiol* 2002; **43**:

229–236.

33. Greenwald JA, McMullen HF, Coppa GF, Newman RM. Standardization of surgeon-controlled variables: impact on outcome in patients with acute cholecystitis. *Ann Surg* 2000; **231**: 339–344.

34. Salman B, Yuksel O, Irkorucu O *et al.* Urgent laparoscopic cholecystectomy is the best management for biliary colic. A prospective randomized study of 75 cases. *Dig Surg* 2005; **22**: 95–99.

35. Robertson GS, Wemyss-Holden SA, Maddern GJ. The best management for 'crescendo biliary colic' is urgent laparoscopic cholecystectomy. *Postgrad Med J* 1998; **74**: 681–682.

36. Barie PS, Eachempati SR. Acute acalculous cholecystitis. *Curr Gastroenterol Report* 2003; **5**: 302–309.

37. Deitch EA, Engel JM. Acute acalculous cholecystitis. Ultrasonic diagnosis. *Am J Surg* 1981; **142**: 290–292.

38. Shaffer EA. Gallbladder sludge: what is its clinical significance? *Curr Gastroenterol Report* 2001; **3**: 166–173.

39. Ko CW, Sekijima JH, Lee SP. Biliary sludge. *Ann Intern Med* 1999; **130**: 301–311.

40. Lee KF, Wong J, Li JC, Lai PB. Polypoid lesions of the gallbladder. *Am J Surg* 2004; **188**: 186–190.

Jake E.J. Krige Stephen J. Beningfield
John M. Shaw

9

Modern management of bleeding oesophageal varices

Normal portal vein pressure ranges from 5–10 mmHg. Portal hypertension occurs when the pressure exceeds 12 mmHg,[1] which results in compensatory porto-systemic venous collateral formation, increased splanchnic blood flow and disturbed intrahepatic circulation.[2] These consequences lead to the important complications of portal hypertension which include variceal bleeding, hepatic encephalopathy, ascites, hepatorenal syndrome, recurrent infection and coagulo-pathy that play a major role in the morbidity and mortality of patients with chronic liver diseases.[3] Oesophagastric varices form part of the collateral venous system that diverts high-pressure portal blood via the left gastric, short gastric and oesophageal perforator veins to the systemic azygous system and are important because of their propensity to bleed with resulting morbidity and mortality.[4] Epigastric and abdominal wall collateral vessels also enlarge with recanalisation of the umbilical vein, and multiple retroperitoneal collaterals may complicate surgical intervention. Splenomegaly and hypersplenism develop because of impeded splenic vein outflow.

AETIOLOGY

Portal hypertension has a wide variety of causes and geographic prevalences.[5] Cirrhosis dominates in the Western world, while schistosomiasis is the most

Jake E.J. Krige MB ChB FACS FRCS(Ed) FCS(SA) (for correspondence)
Medical Research Council Liver Research Centre and Department of Surgery, University of Cape Town Health Sciences Faculty, Anzio Road, Observatory 7925, Cape Town, South Africa
E-mail: jake@curie.uct.ac.za

Stephen J. Beningfield MB ChB FF Rad (D) SA
Division of Radiology, University of Cape Town Health Sciences Faculty, Anzio Road, Observatory 7925, Cape Town, South Africa

John M. Shaw MB BCh FCS(SA)
Department of Surgery, University of Cape Town Health Sciences Faculty, Anzio Road, Observatory 7925, Cape Town, South Africa

Table 1 Causes of portal hypertension

INCREASED RESISTANCE TO BLOOD FLOW
> **Presinusoidal**
>> Extrahepatic
>>> Splenic vein thrombosis
>>> Portal vein thrombosis
>> Intrahepatic
>>> Schistosomiasis
>>> Primary biliary cirrhosis
>>> Sarcoidosis
>>> Congenital hepatic fibrosis
> **Sinusoidal**
>> Cirrhosis
>> Haemochromatosis
>> Wilson's disease
> **Post-sinusoidal**
>> Veno-occlusive disease
>> Budd–Chiari syndrome
>> Right heart failure
>> Constrictive pericarditis

INCREASED PORTAL BLOOD FLOW
> **Increased splenic blood flow**
> **Arterial-portal venous fistula**

common cause world-wide. Two mechanisms lead to portal hypertension: (i) increased portal resistance; and (ii) increased portal inflow. Increased resistance to flow is classified as presinusoidal, sinusoidal and postsinusoidal (Table 1). Presinusoidal obstruction of the portal system generally occurs without hepatocyte dysfunction and has a good prognosis,[6] whereas sinusoidal obstruction, commonly due to alcoholic or hepatitis-related cirrhosis, is associated with decreased hepatocyte function and a poorer long-term outcome. Postsinusoidal hypertension is uncommon and is usually due to the Budd Chiari syndrome.[7]

NATURAL HISTORY

The rational management of oesophageal varices depends on a clear understanding of the risks of bleeding in individual patients, the possibility of subsequent re-bleeding and the likely response to each type of therapy.[8] Although about 90% of patients with cirrhosis will ultimately develop varices, only one-third of compensated and two-thirds of decompensated cirrhotic patients have varices at the time of the initial diagnosis of cirrhosis.[1] The risk of bleeding if varices are present can be predicted by: (i) the presence of large oesophageal varices; (ii) portal pressure over 12 mmHg; and (iii) the degree of liver decompensation. Of patients with varices, 30% will ultimately bleed; of these, one-quarter die as a consequence of the bleeding.[5] There is a 70% chance of subsequent re-bleeding, with a similar mortality.[9]

Table 2 Child's classification of functional liver status

	Number of points		
	1	2	3
Bilirubin (μmol/l)	< 34	34–51	> 51
Albumin (g/l)	> 35	28–35	< 28
Prothrombin time	< 3	3–10	> 10
Ascites	None	Mild	Moderate-to-severe
Encephalopathy	None	Mild	Moderate-to-severe

Grade A, 5–6 points; Grade B, 7–9 points; Grade C, 10–15 points.

Careful assessment of hepatic functional reserve is necessary before selecting the most appropriate treatment.[10] The degree of hepatic decompensation is the most important determinant of long-term survival after a variceal bleed.[11] The Child's grade is a useful scoring system, and is the most practical and widely used predictor of survival (Table 2). In Western countries, variceal bleeding accounts for 7% of all upper gastrointestinal bleeding, although this varies geographically (11% in the US, 5% in the UK), depending on the prevalence of alcoholic liver disease.[10]

Key point 1

- Of patients who have varices, 30% ultimately bleed, of whom one-quarter die as a consequence of the bleeding. There is a 70% chance of subsequent re-bleeding, with a similar mortality.

MANAGEMENT OF ACUTE VARICEAL BLEEDING

CHOICE OF THERAPY

The possibility of variceal bleeding should be considered in all patients who present with upper gastrointestinal bleeding and who have known risk factors for chronic liver disease, or clinical evidence of portal hypertension. The modern management of acute variceal bleeding requires a multidisciplinary approach, as a variety of therapeutic options may have to be used either sequentially or combined in individual patients (Table 3). Several important considerations influence the choice of therapy, as well as the prognosis, in individual patients. These include the natural history of the disease causing the portal hypertension, the site of the bleeding varices, residual hepatic function, the presence of associated systemic disease, continuing alcohol abuse, patency of major splanchnic veins and the response to each specific treatment.[6]

GENERAL STRATEGY

All patients with suspected variceal bleeding require hospitalisation. The immediate aims of emergency treatment involve haemodynamic stabilisation, blood-volume replacement, control of bleeding, support of vital organ function and prevention of complications due to hypovolaemic shock and incipient liver failure.[12] Patients should be nursed in an intensive care or high dependency unit, and standard resuscitation protocols for major gastrointestinal bleeding instituted.[13] Although variceal bleeding stops spontaneously in 60% of patients, it is not possible to predict which patients will continue to bleed.[5] Many patients with acute variceal bleeding have liver decompensation with varying degrees of hepatic encephalopathy, ascites, coagulopathy, bacteraemia and malnutrition, each of which requires specific treatment.[14]

Major variceal bleeding is a life-threatening event and treatment must be rapid, efficient and seamless, as intervention may become increasingly complex if bleeding continues.[6] Patients should be transferred, once stable and adequately resuscitated, to a centre which has all the necessary facilities and expertise as subsequent management may require advanced multidisciplinary

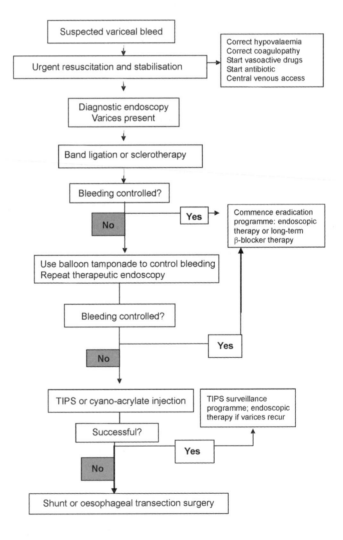

Fig. 1 Algorithm for the management of acute variceal bleeding.

investigations and intervention if bleeding continues or recurs.[5] A suggested management algorithm is shown in Figure 1.

INITIAL MEASURES

The extent and urgency of initial therapy depend on the severity of the bleeding. Establishment and maintenance of a secure airway and prompt resuscitation with restoration of circulating blood volume are vital and precede any diagnostic studies. Intravenous access is obtained via a secure large-bore venous cannula.[6] Central venous access may be required early, preferably after correction of existing coagulopathy. While blood is being cross-matched, crystalloid solution is rapidly infused until the blood pressure is restored and urine output is adequate. However, saline infusions may aggravate ascites and must, therefore, be avoided; overzealous expansion of circulating blood volume may cause a rebound increase in portal pressures and precipitate further bleeding.[15] Central venous pressure should, therefore, be maintained at 2–5 cmH$_2$O. Patients who are haemodynamically unstable, elderly or who have cardiac or pulmonary disease should be monitored using a pulmonary artery catheter because injudicious administration of fluids, combined with vasoactive drugs, may lead to rapid onset of oedema, ascites and hyponatraemia.[8] Clotting factors are often deficient and fresh blood, fresh frozen plasma and vitamin K$_1$ are frequently required.[12] Platelet transfusions may also be necessary. Sedatives should be avoided to prevent worsening of incipient encephalopathy. All patients with cirrhosis and upper gastro-intestinal bleeding should receive short-term prophylactic antibiotics to prevent serious infectious complications.[16]

Key point 2

- Patients who are shocked, elderly or who have cardiac or pulmonary disease should be monitored using a pulmonary artery catheter because injudicious administration of crystalloids, combined with vasoactive drugs, may lead to rapid onset of oedema, ascites and hyponatraemia.

PHARMACOLOGICAL THERAPY

Pharmacological therapy has evolved into an effective first-line treatment in patients with probable variceal bleeding.[17] Empirical pharmacological therapy has a critical advantage in that special technical expertise for administration and monitoring is not required. Most endoscopy units recommend that pharmacological therapy be started when a diagnosis of variceal bleeding is suspected and before emergency endoscopy is performed. This policy has the theoretical advantage of controlling bleeding before the initial endoscopy, which makes both diagnosis and immediate endoscopic therapy easier.[5]

Previously, a continuous intravenous infusion of vasopressin at 0.4 U/min, combined with glyceryl trinitrate (to prevent coronary spasm), was used.[5]

Vasopressin is used less frequently today as newer agents have proven to be superior.[17] Glypressin (terlipressin), the synthetic analogue of vasopressin, has fewer side-effects and has the added advantage of being effective in 2-mg intravenous bolus doses administered 4-hourly, simplifying administration. Early administration of glypressin has shown improved survival.[15]

Somatostatin and its synthetic analogues, octreotide and vapreotide, stop variceal bleeding in up to 80% of patients and, because of their excellent safety profile, can be used without special monitoring. Somatostatin is administered as a continuous intravenous infusion of 250 mg/h, after an initial bolus dose of 250 mg. Octreotide is given as an intravenous infusion of 50 mg/h. β-Blockade is ineffective and contra-indicated in patients who are actively bleeding and are shocked.[6]

EMERGENCY ENDOSCOPY

Urgent endoscopy has a crucial role in the management of portal hypertensive patients with suspected variceal bleeding.[18] Endoscopy is mandatory to confirm that a patient with cirrhosis is indeed bleeding from varices, as up to one-third of portal hypertensive patients may instead be bleeding from non-variceal sources.[5] Patients with varices can usually be separated into three groups: (i) those with active variceal bleeding; (ii) those with variceal bleeding that has stopped; and (iii) those who have varices, but are bleeding from other causes such as a peptic ulcer, Mallory-Weiss tear or portal hypertensive gastropathy.[7]

Any well-trained endoscopist can undertake endoscopic intervention in patients who have oesophageal variceal bleeding.[18] Emergency endoscopy is performed in an endoscopy suite where all the necessary equipment is available. Many units have fully-equipped, mobile, emergency endoscopy trolleys which can be taken, if necessary, into the operating theatre or the intensive care unit. It is imperative that full resuscitative facilities are available, together with skilled support staff experienced in dealing with emergencies. Two endoscopy assistants should be present throughout as careful monitoring is critical during the procedure. Emergency endoscopy should not commence until satisfactory venous access is established, and volume replacement and resuscitation with blood products are initiated to correct hypovolaemia. If bleeding is profuse or if the patient is encephalopathic, endotracheal intubation is essential before endoscopy to protect the airway and avoid aspiration.[5]

Key point 3

- Endoscopy is mandatory to confirm that a patient with cirrhosis is indeed bleeding from varices, as up to one-third of portal hypertensive patients may instead be bleeding from non-variceal sources.

IMMEDIATE ENDOSCOPIC THERAPY

If variceal bleeding is encountered at endoscopy or there is suspicion that varices were the cause of the bleeding, immediate variceal band ligation or sclerotherapy is performed (Fig. 1). If endoscopic intervention is deferred until the next elective endoscopy list in patients who have temporarily stopped bleeding, there is the distinct danger of further major variceal bleeding during the interval period, with consequent morbidity and mortality.[18]

INJECTION SCLEROTHERAPY

In the past, injection sclerotherapy was the most widely used endoscopic treatment. Sclerotherapy has now been replaced by endoscopic variceal band ligation as first-line endoscopic therapy.[19] Sclerotherapy, when used, is performed using a video endoscope and a freehand injection technique, without an oversheath. Any of three different sclerotherapy techniques can be used.[20] Sclerosant may be injected directly into the varices ('intra-variceal') to thrombose the varices, or into the submucosa adjacent to the varices ('para-variceal') to produce submucosal oedema which stops acute variceal bleeding and causes thickening of the overlying mucosa, preventing later bleeding (Fig. 2), or a combined technique.[21] Many endoscopists use the combined para- and intravariceal injection technique for acute variceal bleeding and the intravariceal technique for elective injection, when varices are smaller.[18]

Subsequent sclerotherapy injections are performed at weekly intervals, until all the varices have been eradicated.[22] Once eradication of the varices has been achieved, further endoscopic assessment is performed at 3 months to confirm continued obliteration.[23] Further surveillance evaluations are performed every 6 months for 2 years, and then annually, for life. If recurrent varices are noted at any time, repeat endoscopy and injection are performed at weekly intervals, until the varices have again been eradicated.[19]

Key point 4

- If endoscopic intervention is deferred until the next elective endoscopy list in patients who have temporarily stopped bleeding, there is the distinct danger of further major variceal bleeding during the interval period, with consequent morbidity and mortality risk.

SCLEROSANTS

Several sclerosant solutions are available with different mechanisms of action and varying complication rates.[24] The most commonly used are 5% ethanolamine oleate, 2–5% sodium morrhuate, polidocanol, and sodium tetradecyl sulphate in varying concentrations.[18] Two types of cyanoacrylate tissue adhesives, histocryl and bucrylate, have also been used to treat variceal bleeding.[25] These are effective in acute bleeding, with success rates of 90% following single injections, but because cyanoacrylate hardens rapidly, serious risks of equipment damage by tissue adhesives exist in inexperienced hands.[25] Tissue adhesives are generally reserved for injection of bleeding gastric varices.

The most common local complication after injection sclerotherapy is oesophageal mucosal ulceration which is usually of no major consequence, healing without further problems.[26] Oesophageal strictures are infrequent and respond to endoscopic dilatation.[26] A serious, but uncommon, complication following variceal sclerotherapy is oesophageal perforation, caused by inadvertent intramural injection of sclerosant into the oesophageal wall, rather than into the varix.[25] Pneumonia can occur in patients with acute variceal

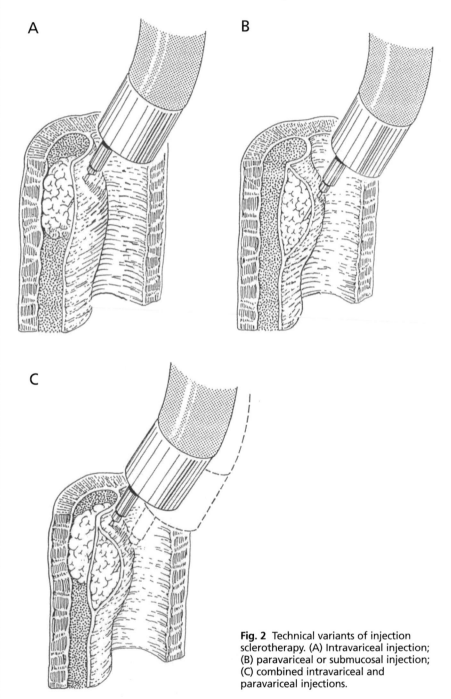

Fig. 2 Technical variants of injection sclerotherapy. (A) Intravariceal injection; (B) paravariceal or submucosal injection; (C) combined intravariceal and paravariceal injections.

bleeding, irrespective of the management used, and may be aggravated by aspiration of blood.[25,26]

OESOPHAGEAL VARICEAL BAND LIGATION

The concept of endoscopic variceal ligation or banding is similar to the technique used for treating haemorrhoids and represents a seminal advance in the endoscopic treatment of varices.[23] Haemostasis is achieved by physical constriction of the varix with a rubber band. Ischaemic necrosis of the strangulated mucosa and submucosa trapped within the band occurs, followed by later sloughing of the banded varix. The resulting shallow mucosal ulcer re-epithelialises after 14–21 days.[27]

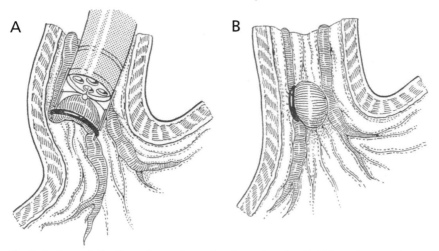

Fig. 3 Endoscopic ligation of oesophageal varices using the flexible endoscope. (A) Varix is identified by the endoscopist. Full contact is made between the end of the ligating device and the varix. Endoscopic suction is applied which results in aspiration of the varix into the ligating device. (B) The draw string is pulled, displacing the stretched elastic band which is released and encircles the neck of the varix, resulting in strangulation and thrombosis.

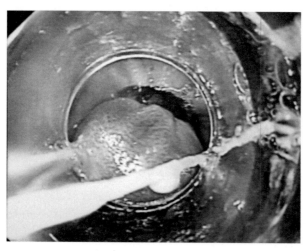

Fig. 4 Rubber band deployed around the base of an oesophageal varix.

Two different types of ligating devices are used. The original single band Stiegmann apparatus places one band at a time, but requires the use of an overtube to allow withdrawal, reloading with a new band and re-insertion of the endoscope. The treatment begins with ligation of the bleeding varix or the most distal part of the target variceal column (Figs 3 and 4). Each column has a single band placed at its lower end. Large varices have additional bands placed more proximally, 2–3 cm higher in the oesophagus.[28] On average, a total of 6–9 bands are applied during the initial session. Repeated banding treatments are performed at 1–2 week intervals until all varices have been eradicated. Progressively fewer bands are required at subsequent sessions as varices decrease in size.[28]

MULTIBAND APPLICATION

The multiband ligator carries 5, 6, 8 or 10 bands (Fig. 5). Each band is separately activated by a draw-string which passes from the ligator through the biopsy channel, and is attached to a trigger unit mounted on the biopsy channel port of the endoscope, which allows sequential firing of the bands.[29] The multiband system obviates the need for an overtube and repeated insertion.[23] The multiband variceal ligator is a significant technical advance over the single shot device; however, because the unit is disposable and cannot be re-used, the current retail cost of $200 per unit may limit the wide-spread use of the multiband device. Complications related to banding are uncommon. Bleeding at an ulcer site after the band has fallen off has been a less frequent complication than that occurring with sclerotherapy ulcers.[28]

Endoscopic variceal ligation is as effective as injection sclerotherapy in the emergency management of bleeding oesophageal varices although blood in the ligating chamber may reduce visibility and make accurate deployment of the bands more difficult. Variceal eradication using ligation requires fewer endoscopic treatment sessions, and causes substantially less local oesophageal complications.[24] Current data demonstrate a clear long-term advantage for ligation in preference to sclerotherapy.[28] Ligation is now regarded as the endoscopic treatment of choice in the management of oesophageal varices.[28]

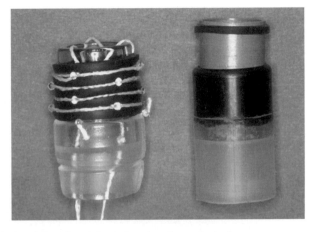

Fig. 5 Loaded multiband and single band endoscopic devices.

Key point 5

- Emergency endoscopic variceal ligation is as effective as injection sclerotherapy for bleeding oesophageal varices and eradicates varices with fewer endoscopic treatment sessions and less complications.

RE-BLEEDING AFTER EMERGENCY ENDOSCOPIC THERAPY

Endoscopic therapy is successful in controlling acute variceal bleeding in over 90% of patients after one or two treatment sessions.[30] Patients who re-bleed after two emergency endoscopy treatments during a single hospital admission have a prohibitively high mortality if further endoscopic therapy is pursued. Such patients should have a balloon tube inserted, be resuscitated and then treated with an alternative method, usually a radiologically placed TIPS stent.

BALLOON TUBE TAMPONADE

Balloon tamponade applies direct mechanical pressure with an inflatable balloon attached to a special nasogastric tube and compresses the varices at the oesophagogastric junction (Fig. 6). A balloon tube is used when emergency endoscopic therapy cannot be safely performed because visibility is obscured by major variceal bleeding, or when patients continue to bleed despite several emergency endoscopic interventions.[8] The balloon tube should always be inserted by experienced staff to avoid complications such as oesophageal perforation or aspiration which may follow incorrect placement. The tube should be left in place for as short a time as possible while the patient is being resuscitated.[5] Recurrent bleeding is common after tube removal, so arrangements must be made to provide skilled endoscopy or alternative therapy. Tube tamponade is a useful rescue procedure as a bridge to more definitive therapy in situations where uncontrolled bleeding occurs.[17]

TECHNIQUE OF BALLOON TUBE INSERTION

Several technical points are important when employing balloon tamponade. Before a balloon tube is inserted in an encephalopathic or comatose patient, the airway must be protected by placing a cuffed endotracheal tube to prevent aspiration. A new balloon tube should always be used, and the balloon pre-tested by inflation under water to exclude leaks. The deflated lubricated balloon tube is passed through a bite-guard via the mouth, after topical pharyngeal anaesthesia. The correct position of the gastric balloon within the stomach must be confirmed by an abdominal radiograph before inflation because inflation of the gastric balloon within the oesophagus may result in oesophageal perforation. Once in position, the balloon is inflated with 50-ml increments of air using a syringe to a total of 250 ml.

The inflated balloon is pulled up to engage snugly and press on the oesophagogastric junction. The balloon is held in place and the tension in the taut tube maintained by using a split tennis ball strapped to the tube at the

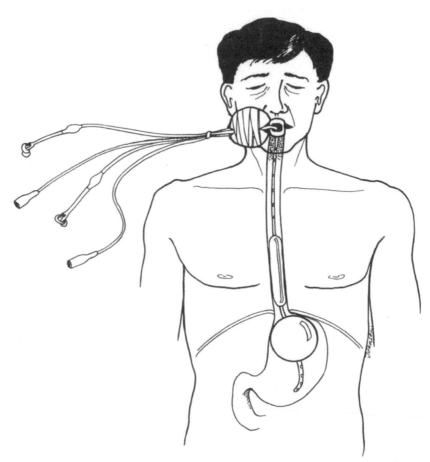

Fig. 6 Four lumen balloon tube. The gastric balloon which is filled with air is held firmly against the oesophagogastric junction by fixing a split tennis ball around the tube at the patient's mouth.

mouth guard which protects the patient's lips from the pressure of the tennis ball (Fig. 6). Inflation of the oesophageal balloon is not usually necessary as traction on the gastric balloon is generally sufficient. If oesophageal balloon inflation is used, a three-way tap and a blood pressure manometer are used to inflate the oesophageal balloon to 40 mmHg and the tube clamped to maintain the balloon pressure. The pressure should be checked regularly and the third lumen, which opens in the oesophagus, placed on constant suction to keep the oesophagus clear of saliva. The gastric lumen is used for either suction or administering medication, such as lactulose.

Patients with a balloon tube in place should be monitored in an intensive care unit as the balloon is uncomfortable and dislodgement by a restless patient may cause complications including injury to the oesophagus or airway obstruction. Once the balloon tube has been inserted and fixed and bleeding has been arrested, resuscitation is continued, clotting defects are corrected, and the patient is made as fit as possible for the necessary subsequent management. The balloon tube should be removed preferably after 6–12 hours, but definitely within 24 hours, to avoid severe oesophageal mucosal ulceration.

Key point 6

- Balloon tubes must always be inserted by experienced staff to avoid complications such as oesophageal perforation or aspiration.

ALTERNATIVE EMERGENCY MANAGEMENT OPTIONS

The main second-line alternatives to first-line pharmacological and endoscopic therapy for acute variceal bleeding are: (i) a radiologically placed transjugular intrahepatic portosystemic shunt (TIPS): (ii) a surgically created portosystemic shunt; or (iii) a staple gun oesophageal transection operation. In patients with recurrent bleeding, a crucial caveat is to identify accurately the cause and site of bleeding, as management differs for injection-induced oesophageal ulceration, recurrent variceal bleeding, gastric varices, and portal hypertensive gastropathy.

Transjugular intrahepatic portosystemic shunt (TIPS)

A TIPS shunt is the emergency procedure of choice for patients in whom endoscopic therapy has failed to stop the bleeding. Until recently, major surgery was the only method of creating a portosystemic shunt. TIPS is a non-operative interventional radiological stent which can be inserted under local anaesthesia. Recent data confirm the utility and efficacy of the TIPS shunt as a salvage procedure for refractory variceal bleeding unresponsive to endoscopic and pharmacological treatment.[31]

In principle, a catheter is inserted into a hepatic vein via a jugular vein puncture. A rigid needle is passed through the catheter and advanced from the right or middle hepatic vein, through a bridge of liver tissue into a major right or left portal vein branch (Fig. 7). After placement of a guide-wire, the tract within the liver tissue is dilated using a 10-mm angioplasty balloon catheter. The communication between the hepatic vein and the portal vein is then held open with an expandable metal stent.[32]

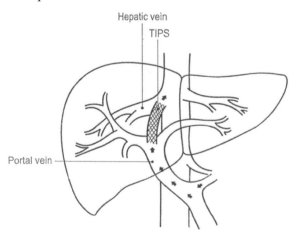

Fig. 7 Transjugular intrahepatic portosystemic shunt. An expandable 10-mm metal stent is placed between a hepatic vein and a portal vein branch.

The major advantage of TIPS stenting is treating failed endoscopic therapy in patients with acute variceal bleeding. The procedure can be performed with low morbidity by an experienced interventional radiologist, even in poor-risk patients. TIPS is an ideal bridge to liver transplantation in patients with acute variceal bleeding, as the procedure maintains the integrity of the porta hepatis and does not alter portal vein anatomy. It is, therefore, preferred by transplant surgeons as the salvage intervention of choice.[33]

Immediate control of variceal bleeding is achieved in over 90% of patients.[32] However, TIPS in uncontrolled variceal bleeding still has a high mortality. Prognosis is poor if patients have developed sepsis, or require inotropic support and ventilation, and have deteriorating liver and renal function.[15] Established renal failure in a decompensated cirrhotic patient with uncontrolled bleeding is a contra-indication to TIPS placement in most units.[32]

Absolute contra-indications to TIPS are polycystic liver disease and right heart failure, while relative contra-indications include portal vein thrombosis, hypervascular liver tumours, and encephalopathy.[32] Disadvantages of the TIPS procedure include the cost (each stent costs about $1000), particularly when more than one procedure is required. Another disadvantage is that, with time, the overall risk of hepatic encephalopathy rate increases to over 30%, a level similar to that with standard portacaval shunts. A further significant problem has been an approximately 50% 1-year occlusion rate, due to pseudo-intimal hyperplasia, often at the hepatic venous end of the shunt. Biliary leaks in the hepatic track are thought to play a role in increasing the risk of occlusion.[33] The introduction of new polytetrafluoroethylene covered stents represent a promising development, with improved primary patency rates and substantially reduced stent dysfunction.

Key point 7

- Renal and liver failure in a cirrhotic patient with uncontrolled bleeding is a contra-indication to TIPS placement.

Surgical options

The need for emergency surgical shunts to control acute variceal bleeding has diminished substantially in the past decade because of the improved efficacy of pharmacological, endoscopic and radiological treatment. While a successful surgical shunt effectively stops acute variceal bleeding and prevents recurrent bleeds, the role of emergency shunting procedures is currently restricted to patients who have failed endoscopic therapy and cannot be salvaged by a TIPS stent for technical reasons. Emergency shunt surgery has an operative mortality greater than 25%, largely determined by the degree of liver decompensation.[34]

A variety of gastric devascularisation and oesophageal transection operations which disconnect the high-pressure portal system from the oesophageal varices have been devised. As a basic principle, the most simple procedure should be used. Oesophageal transection and re-anastomosis using a staple gun, is the preferred emergency procedure for patients in whom endoscopic therapy has failed and when TIPS or an operative shunt are not feasible. Previous sclerotherapy may increase the difficulty and the risk of performing the transection due to sclerosant-induced ulceration and peri-oesophageal fibrosis. Oesophageal transection combined with extensive oesophageal and gastric devascularisation is not justified in the emergency setting.[5]

Four trials have compared sclerotherapy with oesophageal transection after failed medical treatment, and one trial has compared sclerotherapy with portacaval shunt surgery. Failure to control bleeding was higher with sclerotherapy alone while re-bleeding, assessed in three trials, was significantly higher with injection sclerotherapy, although there were no significant differences in mortality.[34]

PREVENTION OF VARICEAL RE-BLEEDING

Although the chances of recurrent variceal bleeding diminish with time, up to 70% of untreated patients will have further variceal bleeding. For this reason, all patients who have had an initial variceal bleed should have long-term management aimed at preventing further bleeding. Once the acute bleeding episode has been controlled and the patient is stabilised, a detailed evaluation must be made to identify the cause of the portal hypertension, its severity and the likely natural history of any underlying liver disease, together with the location and extent of bleeding varices.[10]

The goals of definitive treatment are prevention of further portal hypertensive bleeding while avoiding encephalopathy and liver failure.[6] The choice of definitive therapy is based on the extent of varices, the availability of resources, and local expertise.[6] The treatment options vary in their expense, degree of skill required and likely success. Endoscopic therapy has been established during the past decade as a cornerstone of treatment for the prevention of recurrent oesophageal variceal bleeding.[17]

TREATMENT OPTIONS TO PREVENT RE-BLEEDING

Although endoscopic variceal ligation is preferred in many units as the long-term therapy of choice in most patients, pharmacological treatment with propranolol alone or combined with nitrates is an acceptable alternative long-term therapy in selected patients. Operative shunts, particularly the distal splenorenal shunt (DSRS) and the 8-mm portacaval H-graft have a role in good-risk Child's A or B patients. In Child's C patients with progressively deteriorating synthetic liver function and intractable ascites, liver transplantation becomes an important consideration.

PHARMACOLOGICAL THERAPY

The main goal of pharmacological therapy is to reduce the portal pressure below 12 mmHg which effectively prevents recurrent bleeding. The use of β-blockers as primary long-term therapy has considerable support in the current literature.[35] Several meta-analyses have concluded that β-blockers, principally propranolol, significantly reduce the incidence of recurrent bleeding and improve long-term survival when compared with placebo.[36] The target of therapy with propranolol is to reduce portal pressure, as reflected by the indirect signs of heart rate reduction by 25%, or to 55 beats/min.[3]

Unfortunately, β-blockade has drawbacks. There are several relative contra-indications to β-blockade, including bronchial asthma, chronic obstructive pulmonary disease, peripheral vascular disease, congestive cardiac failure, and unstable insulin-dependent diabetes mellitus. Once treatment is initiated, β-blocker-induced side-effects may also be a problem. The most common side-effects are loss of energy, depression, impotence and headaches. In a minority of patients, these side-effects may be sufficiently severe to cause discontinuation of treatment. Thus, a significant proportion of the population at risk may not be suitable for treatment with β-blockers, or stop taking the drug as a result of side-effects. In addition, one-third of patients treated with standard doses of β-blockers do not have a significant reduction in portal venous pressure.[3]

Where patient compliance is good, long-term propranolol therapy is a viable alternative to endoscopic management of varices. If patients have a recurrent bleed while on adequate propranolol therapy, different treatment, particularly endoscopic therapy, should be instituted. The risk of β-blocker side-effects has led to the evaluation of other drugs to reduce portal pressure. These include nitrates, with isosorbide-5-mononitrate being increasingly used in clinical practice. Other oral medications such as α_2-agonists (e.g. clonidine), calcium-channel antagonists (e.g. verapamil), and serotonin antagonists (e.g. ketanserin), have been evaluated in studies but have not gained wide-spread clinical acceptance.

SURGICAL SHUNTS FOR LONG-TERM CONTROL

The role of surgery in patients who have portal hypertension and bleeding varices has changed dramatically in the last decade. While the use of surgical shunts has markedly reduced, liver transplantation as a treatment has continued to grow. Portosystemic shunts are classified as non-selective, selective, or partial, depending on how much hepatic portal flow is preserved. Non-selective shunts decompress the entire portal system by diverting all portal blood flow. Selective shunts attempt to decompress only the variceal-bearing compartment of the portal venous system while preserving some portal flow to the liver. Partial shunts, in contrast, incompletely decompress the portal system and maintain some portal flow.[34]

Total non-selective end-to-side or side-to-side portacaval shunts effectively control acute variceal bleeding and prevent recurrent bleeding and were the gold standard in the past. However, these total decompression shunts are associated with severe, unpredictable and often incapacitating side-effects, particularly encephalopathy and deteriorating liver function due to diminished prograde portal perfusion with the result that total portosystemic shunts are seldom used now. All shunts are major operations, especially in poor-risk patients and carry significant morbidity and mortality of up to 20% in reputable recent series, even as elective procedures.[34]

A widely used selective shunt for long-term management has been the distal splenorenal shunt (DSRS). A DSRS should be considered for patients who have well-preserved liver function, who do not have readily available tertiary care, including repeated endoscopic therapy, or who are unlikely to be compliant with follow-up. This shunt has the theoretical advantage of selectively shunting left upper quadrant portal venous blood away from the oesophagogastric varices, while preserving superior mesenteric and portal blood flow to the liver. Although prograde flow tends to diminish with time due to recollateralisation, this shunt has a lower encephalopathy rate than standard portacaval shunts in non-alcoholic patients. The disadvantages of the DSRS are the complexity and technical difficulty of the operation, with increased blood loss, operating time and morbidity, as well as late shunt occlusion, ascites and portal vein thrombosis. DSRS is, nonetheless, an effective shunt for patients who have recurrent variceal bleeding despite pharmacological and endoscopic treatment and are good surgical candidates, with good synthetic liver function, no history of pancreatitis and no ascites. DSRS are not used in patients with refractory ascites or Child C patients with poor hepatic function.[6] In a randomised trial, DSRS and TIPS were equally effective in Child A and B patients with refractory variceal bleeding.[37] There was no significant difference in re-bleeding rates (6% after DSRS and 9% after TIPS), encephalopathy or survival, but TIPS patients required significantly more re-interventions.[37]

Partially decompressing shunts, such as side-to-side calibrated shunts or small diameter prosthetic mesocaval or H-graft portacaval shunts maintain a degree of portal perfusion, while reducing portal pressure. The narrow-diameter 8-mm prosthetic PTFE H-graft portacaval shunt (PCS) is an effective alternative to the distal splenorenal shunt, has recurrent bleeding rates of less than 10%, new onset encephalopathy is uncommon, and pre-existing ascites usually improves. Data from a randomised trial show that the 8-mm H-graft PCS provides more reliable partial portal decompression than TIPS, with less recurrent shunt stenosis or thrombosis, but up to a quarter of patients lose hepatoportal flow, especially in those with advanced cirrhosis.[38] Indeed, the longer the follow-up after shunting, the more likely the finding of reversed hepatoportal flow. The surgical shunt performed better for control of bleeding, reduced the need for transplant, and improved overall shunt success rate, although survival was not significantly different.[38]

DEVASCULARISATION AND TRANSECTION OPERATIONS

Although oesophageal transection alone was previously used in the management of acute variceal bleeding, more extensive gastric and oesophageal devascularisation operations with transection of the lower oesophagus have also been used in some centres for long-term management. These major procedures are particularly popular in Japan.[7] The Sugiura procedure which incorporates an oesophagogastric devascularisation with splenectomy and preservation of the coronary and para-oesophageal veins has a re-bleeding rate of less than 10% in Japanese series. Modifications of this procedure have not been as successful in the West, probably due to a difference in the proportion of patients with alcoholic cirrhosis. The Sugiura procedure is useful in patients who are unable to undergo shunting because of extensive portal, splenic, and superior mesenteric vein thrombosis. Controlled trials have shown that, although they are as effective as repeated endoscopic therapy, long-term endoscopic therapy is simpler and less costly.[1] Devascularisation and transection procedures are now reserved for patients with recurrent variceal bleeding despite endoscopic and pharmacological treatment who are not candidates for TIPS and have venous vasculature unsuitable for shunt operations.

LIVER TRANSPLANTATION

Liver transplantation is the only definitive treatment that both cures the underlying liver disease and eradicates portal hypertension.[7] All patients who have variceal bleeding and significant liver decompensation should be considered for hepatic transplantation, even though only a small percentage of patients will ultimately undergo transplantation. In potential transplant candidates with acute variceal bleeding, emergency endoscopic therapy is the treatment of choice. If endoscopic therapy fails to control active variceal bleeding and if a donor liver is not immediately available, an emergency TIPS procedure should be performed as a salvage procedure to control bleeding before transplantation. Once the patient has recovered from the acute variceal bleed, early transplantation should be performed if further evaluation confirms that the patient is a suitable liver transplant candidate. It is end-stage liver disease, rather than variceal bleeding, that dictates the need for such surgery, which treats both portal hypertension and variceal bleeding with the additional advantage of restoring liver function. Transplant is the ultimate 'shunt'. Long-term survival in established liver transplant units now exceeds 70%. Unfortunately, transplantation is not available to many patients because of alcohol recidivism, lack of patient compliance, geographic constraints, donor pool access and post-transplant risks of immunosuppression and infection. Patients with good liver function who require surgery should be considered for a distal splenorenal shunt or H-graft, and not a transplant.

Key point 8

- Liver transplantation is the only treatment that cures the underlying liver disease and eradicates portal hypertension.

CONCLUSIONS

The range of treatment options for bleeding oesophageal varices has expanded markedly during the past two decades. Increasingly sophisticated methods of management have developed in response to the evolving understanding of the pathophysiological processes underlying portal hypertension. In particular, the introduction of safer variceal endotherapy in the form of banding, the refinement of the radiological TIPS procedure with the prospect of better results with covered stents, and improved survival after liver transplantation have had a significant impact on treatment and survival. Endoscopic treatment has become the principal first-line intervention in patients with bleeding oesophageal varices, both during the acute event, and for long-term prevention of recurrent bleeding. Emergency surgical procedures are seldom indicated. The treatment of both acute and persistent recurrent variceal bleeding is best accomplished by an experienced, knowledgeable, and well-equipped team using a multidisciplinary integrated approach.[34] Optimal management should provide the full spectrum of treatment options including pharmacological therapy, endoscopic treatment, interventional radiological procedures, surgical shunts and liver transplantation.

Key points for clinical practice

- Of patients who have varices, 30% ultimately bleed, of whom one-quarter die as a consequence of the bleeding. There is a 70% chance of subsequent re-bleeding, with a similar mortality.

Patients who are shocked, elderly or who have cardiac or pulmonary disease should be monitored using a pulmonary artery catheter because injudicious administration of fluids, combined with vasoactive drugs may lead to rapid onset of oedema, ascites and hyponatraemia.

Endoscopy is mandatory to confirm that a patient with cirrhosis is indeed bleeding from varices, as up to one-third of portal hypertensive patients may instead be bleeding from non-variceal sources.

If endoscopic intervention is deferred until the next elective endo-scopy list in patients who have temporarily stopped bleeding, there is the distinct danger of further major variceal bleeding during the interval period, with consequent morbidity and mortality.

Emergency endoscopic variceal ligation is as effective as injection sclerotherapy for bleeding oesophageal varices and eradicates varices with fewer endoscopic treatment sessions and less complications.

Balloon tubes must always be inserted by experienced staff to avoid complications such as oesophageal perforation or aspiration.

Renal and liver failure in a cirrhotic patient with uncontrolled bleeding is a contra-indication to TIPS placement.

Liver transplantation is the only treatment that cures the underlying liver disease and eradicates portal hypertension.

References

1. D'Amico G, Pagliaro L, Bosch J. The treatment of portal hypertension: a meta-analytic review. *Hepatology* 1995; **22**: 332–354.
2. Krige JE, Beckingham IJ. Portal hypertension: varices. *BMJ* 2001; **322**: 348–351.
3. Bosch J, Abraldes JG, Groszmann R. Current management of portal hypertension. *J Hepatol* 2003; **38**: S54–S58.

4. Garcia-Tsao G. Current management of the complications of cirrhosis and portal hypertension: variceal hemorrhage, ascites, and spontaneous bacterial peritonitis. *Gastroenterology* 2001; **120**: 726–748.

5. Bornman PC, Krige JEJ, Terblanche J. Management of oesophageal varices. *Lancet* 1994; **343**: 1079–1084.

6. Rosemurgy AS, Zervos EE. Management of variceal hemorrhage. *Curr Probl Surg* 2003; **40**: 263–343.

7. Wright AS, Rikkers LF. Current management of portal hypertension. *J Gastrointest Surg* 2005; **9**: 992–1005.

8. Krige JEJ, Beningfield SJ, Bornman PC. Liver and portal circulation. In: Burnand K, Young A, Rowlands BJ, Scholfield J, Lucas J. (eds) *New AIRD'S Textbook of Surgery*, 3rd edn. London: Churchill Livingstone, 2005.

9. Gow PJ, Chapman RW. Modern management of oesophageal varices. *Postgrad Med J* 2001; **77**: 75–81.

10. Krige JEJ, Beckingham IJ. Portal hypertension – 1: varices. In: *ABC of Liver, Pancreas and Gallbladder*. London: British Medical Journal Publishing Group, 2001; 18–21.

11. de Franchis R. Evaluation and follow-up of patients with cirrhosis and oesophageal varices. *J Hepatol* 2003; **38**: 361–363.

12. Lubel JS, Angus PW. Modern management of portal hypertension. *Intern Med J* 2005; **35**: 45–49.

13. Nietsch HH. Management of portal hypertension. *J Clin Gastroenterol* 2005; **39**: 232–236.

14. Zaman A, Chalasani N. Bleeding caused by portal hypertension. *Gastroenterol Clin North Am* 2005; **34**: 623–642.

15. Mihas AA, Sanyal AJ. Recurrent variceal bleeding despite endoscopic and medical therapy. *Gastroenterology* 2004; **127**: 621–629.

16. de Franchis R. Evolving consensus in portal hypertension. Report of the Baveno IV consensus workshop on methodology of diagnosis and therapy in portal hypertension. *J Hepatol* 2005; **43**: 167–176.

17. Sharara AI, Rockey DC. Gastroesophageal variceal hemorrhage. *N Engl J Med* 2001; **345**: 669–681.

18. Krige JE, Bornman PC. Endoscopic treatment of oesophageal varices. *S Afr J Surg* 2000; **38**: 82–88.

19. Terblanche J, Krige JEJ. Endoscopic therapy in the management of esophageal varices: injection sclerotherapy and variceal ligation. In: Nyhus N, Baker B, Fischer M. (eds) *Mastery of Surgery*, 4th edn. New York: Lippincott, Williams, Wilkins. 2001; 1388–1402.

20. Krige JEJ, Terblanche J. Injection sclerotherapy of oesophageal varices. In: Jamieson GG, DeBas HT. (eds) *Rob and Smith's Operative Surgery. Surgery of the Upper Gastrointestinal Tract*, 5th edn. London: Chapman and Hall Medical, 1994; 10–20.

21. Krige JEJ, Terblanche J. Injection sclerotherapy of oesophageal varices. In: Carter D, Russell RCG, Pitt H, Bismuth H. (eds) *Rob and Smith's Operative Surgery. Surgery of the Liver, Pancreas and Bile Ducts*, 5th edn. London: Chapman and Hall Medical, 1996; 163–172.

22. Krige JEJ, Kotze UK, Bornman PC, Shaw JM, Klipin M. Recurrence, rebleeding and survival after endoscopic injection sclerotherapy in alcoholic patients with bleeding esophageal varices. *Ann Surg* 2006; **244**: 764–770.

23. Terblanche J, Stiegmann G, Krige JEJ, Bornman PC. Long-term management of variceal bleeding: The place of varix injection and ligation. *World J Surg* 1994; **18**: 185–192.

24. Krige JEJ, Shaw JM, Bornman PC. The evolving role of endoscopic treatment for bleeding esophageal varices. *World J Surg* 2005; **29**: 966–973.

25. Krige JEJ, Bornman PC, Shaw JM, Apostolou C. Complications of endoscopic variceal therapy. *S Afr J Surg* 2005; **43**: 177–194.

26. Krige JEJ, Bornman PC, Terblanche J. Complications of sclerotherapy. In: Sivak MV. (ed) *Gastrointestinal Endoscopy*, 2nd edn. New York: WB Saunders, 2000; 860–876.

27. Krige JEJ, Botha JF, Bornman PC. Endoscopic variceal ligation for bleeding esophageal varices. *Dig Endosc* 1999; **11**: 315–320.

28. Tait IS, Krige JEJ, Terblanche J. Endoscopic band ligation of oesophageal varices. *Br J Surg* 1999; **86**: 437–446.

29. Krige JEJ, Terblanche J. Endoscopic sclerotherapy and variceal band ligation in the management of bleeding esophageal varices. In: Blumgart L, Fong Y. (eds) *Surgery of the*

Liver and Bile Ducts, 3rd edn. Baltimore, MD: WB Saunders, 2000; 1885–1906.

30. Krige JEJ, Bornman PC, Goldberg PA, Terblanche J. Variceal rebleeding and recurrence after endoscopic injection sclerotherapy: a prospective evaluation in 204 patients. *Arch Surg* 2000; **135**: 1315–1322.

31. McAvoy NC, Hayes PC. The use of transjugular intrahepatic portosystemic stent shunt in the management of acute oesophageal variceal haemorrhage. *Eur J Gastroenterol Hepatol* 2006; **18**: 1135–1141.

32. Boyer TD, Haskal ZJ. The role of transjugular intrahepatic portosystemic shunt in the management of portal hypertension. *Hepatology* 2005; **41**: 386–400.

33. Boyer TD. Transjugular intrahepatic portosystemic shunt: current status. *Gastroenterology* 2003; **124**: 1700–1710.

34. Knechtle SJ, Rikkers LF. Current management of esophageal variceal bleeding. *Adv Surg* 1999; **33**: 439–458.

35. Bosch J, Garcia-Pagan JC. Prevention of variceal rebleeding. *Lancet* 2003; **361**: 952–954.

36. Samonakis DN, Triantos CK, Thalheimer U, Patch DW, Burroughs AK. Management of portal hypertension. *Postgrad Med J* 2004; **80**: 634–641.

37. Henderson JM, Boyer TD, Kutner MH *et al.* and DIVERT Study Group. Distal splenorenal shunt versus transjugular intrahepatic portal systematic shunt for variceal bleeding: a randomized trial. *Gastroenterology* 2006; **130**: 1643–1651.

38. Rosemurgy AS, Bloomston M, Clark WC, Thometz DP, Zervos EE. H-graft portacaval shunts versus TIPS: ten-year follow-up of a randomized trial with comparison to predicted survivals. *Ann Surg* 2005; **241**: 238–246.

Malcolm A. Loudon

10

Haemorrhoid surgery: what is best practice?

Haemorrhoids consist of vascular cushions that are intimately involved in the maintenance of continence and discrimination between flatus and faeces. These cushions are normally maintained in position by the suspensory ligaments.[1] The most widely supported theory is that symptomatic haemorrhoids result from disruption of these ligaments permitting downward prolapse of the cushions into and beyond the anal canal during defaecation. This prolapse results in constriction of the haemorrhoids between the faecal bolus and the ring of the sphincter mechanism. As a consequence, swelling due to vascular engorgement occurs with a sensation of fullness and bleeding being common symptoms. While initially spontaneous reduction is the norm, over time patients may find it necessary to reduce their haemorrhoids manually. This is a key symptom in defining the need for formal surgical intervention.

Key point 1

- Manual reduction of haemorrhoids is a strong indication for surgical treatment. Ask the patient if they manually reduce.

With further chronicity, permanent prolapse may occur. This situation results in the other common haemorrhoidal symptoms of mucus seepage with difficulties in hygiene and pruritis, loss of discrimination and continence to flatus or even mild faecal incontinence.

CULTURAL CONSIDERATIONS

Surgical intervention for haemorrhoids is partly determined by patient and cultural considerations. Rates of surgery for haemorrhoids vary from 35/100,000

Malcolm A. Loudon MD ChB FRCSEd(Gen)
Consultant Colorectal and General Surgeon, Aberdeen Royal Infirmary, Aberdeen AB25 2ZN, UK
E-mail: malcolml@doctors.org.uk

in the UK to 50–60/100,000 population/year in the US[2] with higher rates in Italy and Germany. The reasons for such variation include patient perception of symptom severity and cosmesis as well as the historical belief, not unfounded, that surgery is extremely painful. When these factors are considered together with variations in the perception by surgeons of the place for haemorrhoidectomy as an effective treatment and its timing in relationship to the natural history of the disease, such widely varied rates of intervention can be more readily understood.

GRADING OF HAEMORRHOIDS

A number of clinical grading scales are in use. The most widely accepted system is:

Grade I	Never prolapse;
Grade II	Prolapse on defaecation, spontaneously reduce;
Grade III	Prolapse on defaecation, require manual reduction;
Grade IV	Permanent prolapse.

SYMPTOMS

There is a broad correlation between symptoms and grade of haemorrhoids. Bleeding alone, associated with defaecation is generally the main presentation of Grade I haemorrhoids. Grade II haemorrhoids bleed but may also give rise to problems of discrimination between flatus and fluid faeces and contribute to pruritis. Grade III haemorrhoids bleed, sometimes sufficiently to soil underclothing and unrelated to defaecation. In addition, they may cause throbbing discomfort pruritis and difficulty with hygiene. Grade IV haemorrhoids are associated with all of the above; however, problems with discrimination and continence and cleanliness can be severe.

TYPICAL HAEMORRHOIDAL SYMPTOMS
Bleeding
Typically bright red drips into the pan, seen on the paper, covers stool or 'squirts'. Associated with a normal or hard stool and is generally painless.

Prolapse
Patient aware of 'something coming down' or fullness. May reduce spontaneously or require manual reduction.

Pain
Severe pain is in fact unusual unless associated with acutely prolapsed thrombosed haemorrhoids. Most patients do not experience more than throbbing discomfort and more severe pain should alert the surgeon to other possible conditions including anal fissure or sepsis. Unremitting pain associated with bleeding particularly in middle-aged patients raises the possibility of anorectal malignancy.

Problems of discrimination
Due to the prolapse of the haemorrhoidal cushions and their intimate involvement in the continence mechanism, failure to discriminate between gas and faeces can result in considerable social embarrassment.

Soiling

Prolapse of the haemorrhoidal cushions and mucosa results in soiling of perianal skin this, in turn, results in pruritis.

Pruritis

As a result of soiling and difficulties in hygiene aggravated by the external component, faecal material accumulates on perianal skin and may cause severe itch often complicated by secondary yeast infection and development of the itch-scratch-itch cycle.

INDICATIONS FOR INTERVENTION

The decision to intervene, in particular by surgery, should be driven by the impact of symptoms on quality of life. It is important to question the patient directly regarding the nature of their symptoms. Some important indications for operative treatment, particularly soiling and manual reduction are not generally spontaneously volunteered. Manual reduction is a strong indication for surgery as such haemorrhoids are unlikely to respond to dietary measures or minor interventions such as banding.

Key point 2 & 3

- The need for surgical treatment is largely driven by the effect of symptoms on quality of life.
- Important symptoms such as the need to reduce the haemorrhoids manually or soiling may not be readily volunteered.

DIFFERENTIAL DIAGNOSIS

The most important differential diagnosis to exclude is anorectal malignancy. Although inflammatory bowel disease generally presents with severe diarrhoea and the passage of blood and mucopus, anorectal Crohn's disease along with minor anorectal conditions such as fissure *in ano* may be mistaken for haemorrhoids by both patients and less experienced medical practitioners. This is particularly the case if the patient is not adequately examined.

INVESTIGATION

The need for investigation is guided by the presenting symptoms and the risk profile of the patient. In patients under the age of 45 years who present with bright red rectal bleeding as described above, with no adverse family history of colorectal cancer, particularly when associated with other haemorrhoidal symptoms such as pruritis, it is reasonable to confine investigation to digital rectal examination proctoscopy and sigmoidoscopy. The author would strongly advocate the use of the flexible sigmoidoscope following an enema. Many such patients can be seen at direct access or one-stop rectal bleeding clinics. More extensive investigation by endoscopy or radiological imaging may be indicated on clinical grounds, *e.g.* significant anaemia, major alteration in bowel habit, *etc.*

Selective use of ultrasound and anorectal physiology is appropriate particularly in women with a relevant obstetric history but also if there is a history suggestive of sphincter damage including surgical injury. Provided no other pathology is identified, the haemorrhoids should be treated as described previously.

Key point 4 & 5

- Flexible sigmoidoscopy is strongly recommended as a minimum in the investigation of patients with rectal bleeding.

- Endo-anal ultrasound and anorectal physiology assessment is recommended in cases with a previous history suggesting obstetric trauma or iatrogenic injury.

NON-OPERATIVE APPROACHES

CONSERVATIVE MANAGEMENT

This is appropriate for most patients with Grade I and II haemorrhoids. Measures largely include fibre supplementation[3] and increased fluid intake. The patient should be actively encouraged to drink 2–3 litres of water or equivalent fluid each day. While dietary modification may be sufficient, occupational and social considerations may be such that this alone is impractical and fibre supplementation in the form of methylcellulose or isphagula husk may be required. Patients should be encouraged to respond to a call to stool and avoid pronged straining. This may also involve education, for example, discouraging patients from reading in the toilet. Loss of weight may also be of benefit by reducing intra-abdominal pressure.

A minority of patients with more advanced grades of haemorrhoids, who are unsuitable for surgery as a result of co-morbidity or age, may also be suitable only for conservative management in an attempt to minimise symptoms.

OUT-PATIENT TREATMENTS

A myriad of techniques have been used in the out-patient setting. Only two are in general use – rubber band ligation and sclerosant injection;[4] both share a high recurrence rate[5–7] when objectively measured and rarely are subject to severe complications including life-threatening sepsis. Nevertheless, it remains normal colorectal practice in the UK to employ such techniques initially for Grade II and even some Grade III haemorrhoids.

OPERATIVE APPROACHES

EXCISIONAL HAEMORRHOIDECTOMY

The two main techniques in current use are the Milligan and Morgan procedure[8] popular in the UK and Northern Europe and the Ferguson technique[9] which is more popular in the US. The surgical techniques and their variations are widely described.

Both procedures aim to abolish symptoms by excising the primary haemorrhoids while preserving adequate mucocutaneous bridges between the pedicles to prevent anal stenosis.

The most common short-term complication of these procedures is severe pain although less commonly significant early, or more rarely secondary, postoperative haemorrhage may occur. Recent studies have focused on using novel dissection techniques such as laser scalpels and the use of linear cutter stapling devices in the excision of the haemorrhoids. There is, however, little objective evidence to support the superiority of such technology with its greater expense in improving early postoperative outcomes.

Postoperative pain is best dealt with by a multimodality approach and should begin with pre-operative counselling and possibly analgesia at that stage. A package of measures including long-acting local or caudal anaesthesia, non-constipating analgesia, laxatives and, perhaps most importantly, oral metronidazole,[10,11] which has been demonstrated as highly effective in reducing pain and shortening the duration of incapacity. The calcium channel antagonist diltiazem, by relaxing the involuntary sphincter, may provide further reduction in pain.[12]

Key point 6

- Metronidazole is the most important agent in reducing pain after haemorrhoid surgery.

OPEN OR CLOSED TECHNIQUE?

Most previous trials have failed to demonstrate any significant differences in results between patients having their wounds left open and those having them closed. A number of studies demonstrated that many patients having their wounds closed suffered dehiscence as a result of infection. One recent paper reporting a well-conducted, randomised, controlled trial demonstrated overall superiority for the closed Ferguson technique compared with an open Milligan and Morgan haemorrhoidectomy group.[13] This was particularly the case for continence at 1 year with a highly significant result in favour of the closed group. The observation that metronidazole reduces infection and associated pain may appears to have resulted, as in this trial, in its wide-spread use which may have contributed to the trend of recent studies to demonstrate benefit in closing the haemorrhoidectomy wounds.

NON-EXCISIONAL TECHNIQUES

STAPLED HAEMORRHOIDOPEXY

The main change in the surgical approach to haemorrhoids in the past 10 years has been the development of the stapling procedure for haemorrhoids devised by Longo.[14] Unfortunately, a variety of names have been attached including circular anopexy, stapled anoplasty, procedure for prolapse and haemorrhoids (PPH) and stapled haemorrhoidopexy. What the procedure most certainly is not is a stapled haemorrhoidectomy. The author prefers the term stapled haemorrhoidopexy, as agreed by an international working group of surgeons experienced in the procedure,[15] as this most accurately defines the surgical intent of the procedure.

Stapled haemorrhoidopexy approaches the problem of prolapsing haemorrhoids from the standpoint that the prolapse occurs as a result of stretching or disruption of the suspensory ligaments. By excising a ring of mucosa in the distal rectum, the haemorrhoidal cushions are lifted back into their anatomical position. The procedure, therefore, reduces or prevents the constriction of the haemorrhoids by the sphincter mechanism during defaecation. There is probably also reduction in blood flow into the cushions. Finally, as the tissues around the scar mature, the staple line becomes fixed and will tend to prevent prolapse.

Technique

A detailed description of the technique is beyond the scope of this chapter. Briefly, the patient is positioned either in the prone jack-knife position (which the author strongly recommends) or lithotomy position. A prolene purse string suture is placed around 3 cm above the dentate line using a disposable circular anal dilator (CAD), obturator and anoscope. Great care is taken to ensure a good reduction of the prolapse prior to commencing the purse string suture. It is important to ensure that the entire circumference of the mucosa is incorporated. In order to achieve this, particularly where the mucosal prolapse is substantial, the anoscope must be withdrawn and re-inserted between suture bites rather than simply rotated. Once the purse string is complete, the specially designed circular stapler is inserted fully opened through the CAD following the withdrawal of the anoscope. The tails of the suture are then brought through one of the apertures in the housing and gently tensioned. It is imperative to ensure the anvil has passed fully through the suture line as indicated by a palpable 'give'. It is not necessary to tie the suture around the anvil as originally described or to tie the suture outside the housing. Tension is maintained until the stapler is fully closed and fired. Following withdrawal, the donut is checked. It is our policy to send the specimen routinely for histological examination. The donut length will vary according to the degree of prolapse asymmetry at different points. Occasionally, a small defect may be seen in the donut but provided care has been taken to incorporate the full rectal circumference as described above the staple line will be complete on checking and a good functional result is the norm. The staple line is inspected and more often than not two or three absorbable haemostatic sutures are inserted. These may contribute to the effect of the procedure by interrupting the haemorrhoidal vessels. Haemostasis must be obsessive and it is worthwhile observing the staple line for some minutes even when it appears dry. This policy has resulted in a current cumulative incidence of significant postoperative bleeding rate of less than 0.5% in our hands and these results have been replicated in several large series.[16]

SELECTIVE HAEMORRHOIDAL ARTERY LIGATION

Under Doppler ultrasound guidance, the terminal branches of the haemorrhoidal vessels are suture ligated at up to six identified locations. While there are a number of enthusiasts[17,18] for this technique, it is yet to gain wide currency. Reported rates of recurrence seem high.[19]

RESULTS OF SURGERY

Varying rates of satisfaction are reported for all excisional procedures and appear to reflect patient selection and variation in surgical technique. Satisfaction rates of around 80% are reported[20] by some although others have been more cautionary,[21,22] particularly with regard to the incidence of recurrent symptoms. Robust, long-term, outcome measures are also limited in many series by loss of patients from follow-up or limited returns in questionnaire-based studies. Other factors which influence the perceived outcomes of surgery are the particular symptoms sought and while effective in reducing or abolishing bleeding surgery may be less effective in improving continence. Some studies, indeed, appear to demonstrate new continence problems following surgery, possibly as a result of iatrogenic sphincter injury. The stapled technique is consistently superior for early pain and return to activity;[23] reasonable length follow-up suggests that initial control of symptoms is sustained.[24,25] Excisional surgery remains associated with time away from work of 10–34 days for either of the main techniques.

COMPLICATIONS

All interventions for haemorrhoids beyond conservative and dietary measures have been associated with complications. Pain bleeding and urinary retention are common and, on occasion, may be severe. Impotence has been reported following sclerotherapy.[26] Life-threatening sepsis may also occur[27,28] and had raised concerns with particular regard to stapled haemorrhoidopexy.[29] A recent systematic review has confirmed that such devastating complications, while rare, have been associated with all forms of intervention.[30]

There is a suggestion that the majority of cases reported with stapled haemorrhoidopexy have been associated with technical errors such as repeated firing of staplers as a result of incomplete mucosal donut or incorporation of the rectovaginal septum. It is strongly recommended that, in the event of identifying a very incomplete donut after firing of the stapling device, the staple line be carefully inspected and any defects repaired. No further attempts should be made to repeat the procedure with a new purse string and stapler at that stage. This finding is, in fact, unusual and it appears that problems are associated with ill-judged attempts to place further purse string sutures and use further stapling devices. In the relatively uncommon event of a poor result, the procedure can be repeated at a later stage.

Life-threatening sepsis may be heralded by severe pelvic and low abdominal pain together with urinary difficulties. Early imaging by way of computed tomography is recommended and an aggressive surgical policy including defunctioning and radical debridement recommended, particularly if tissue necrosis has developed.

It remains conjecture that the benefit of oral peri-operative metronidazole in the reduction of infection-related postoperative pain might also extend to a reduction in the risk from severe sepsis.

> **Key point 7 & 8**
>
> - All forms of operative intervention have rarely been associated with serious complications.
>
> - The presence of urinary difficulty associated with pelvic or lower abdominal pain and fever raises the problem of potentially life-threatening sepsis following haemorrhoid surgery.

DAY-CASE SURGERY

Traditionally, surgery for haemorrhoids has been perceived, probably correctly, as extremely painful. Traditional adjuncts to treatment such as the placement of non-absorbable packs probably increased, rather than reduced, pain. Until a few years ago, all excisional procedures were carried out as in-patient procedures in most units. Because of the pain associated with the first passage of stool, patients frequently remained in hospital for 3–5 days 'until their bowels moved'. Pressure on hospital beds together with technical changes and improved peri-operative analgesia mean that it is now common to practice haemorrhoid surgery on a day-case or '23-hour' admission basis.

CRITERIA FOR DAY-CASE HAEMORRHOID SURGERY

The usual day-case criteria apply. ASA grade should be no higher than 3. Patients with body mass index greater than 35 kg/m^2 require careful consideration and some anaesthetists will be unhappy about operating on the obese in the prone jack-knife position. Social considerations include reasonable journey time from hospital, access to a telephone and the presence of a responsible adult at home on discharge.

Good pre-operative counselling is essential. Patients should be warned to expect a degree of discomfort for several days and the importance of the early and regular use of analgesics advised during this time. Surgery early in the day is sensible as any early postoperative haemorrhage can be identified and addressed prior to discharge. It is important to emphasise the early and regular

Table 1 Requirements for day-case haemorrhoid surgery

- Patient selection according to standard day-case medical and social criteria
- Adequate pre-operative counselling
- No bowel preparation
- Non-constipating analgesia
- Local anaesthetic agents/caudal block
- Bulking agents
- Topical calcium channel blocker (diltiazem 2%)or nitrate (glyceryl trinitrate 0.2%)
- Metronidazole

use of postoperative analgesia as pain prevention is always easier than abolition of severe postoperative pain. Pretreatment with a non-steroidal anti-inflammatory and intra-operative intravenous paracetamol seem particularly effective in reducing postoperative pain. With such measures, day-case surgery is perfectly feasible in the majority of cases.[31,32] We have previously reported our experience of day-case haemorrhoid surgery[33] and currently achieve day-surgery rates of 80% for all comers and over 90% for socially and physically suitable patients. The requirements for day-case haemorrhoid surgery are summarised in Table 1.

Key point 9

- Patients can safely undergo day-case haemorrhoid surgery subject to the same medical and social criteria as for other procedures.

LONG-TERM COMPLICATIONS AND THEIR TREATMENT

With careful patient selection and high-quality surgery, long-term serious complications from surgical treatment should be uncommon. Sphincter injury may occur with either the excisional haemorrhoidectomy techniques or stapled haemorrhoidopexy. It is important when re-assessing a patient with 'recurrent' haemorrhoidal symptoms to revisit the history carefully. For example, further interventions in a patient who may in the past have undergone Lord's anal dilatation followed by formal haemorrhoidectomy complaining of soiling may be injudicious and certainly should not be undertaken without formal assessment of the sphincter mechanism by ultrasound and manometry.

Anal stenosis following excisional surgery results from overzealous surgery with inadequate preservation of mucocutaneous bridges. This may be severe and occasionally requires flap repair or split skin grafting. A form of distal rectal stenosis is also occasionally seen after stapled haemorrhoidopexy but this is simply treated by gentle dilatation with a proctoscope usually in the out-patient setting. Occasionally, a second dilatation is required.

Two specific complications of stapled haemorrhoidopexy occur. A persistent sensation of urgency and tenesmus lasting several months occurs in a minority usually of male patients. In the extreme form, symptoms can be disabling; however, the condition responds well to treatment with oral nifedipine.[34] A second syndrome of persistent bleeding, usually small volume, is associated with failure of some of the staples to either discharge or to become incorporated in the rectal mucosa. When the patient is examined, a granulomatous appearance is seen in relation to the residual staples. Staple removal resolves the problem.

Key point 9

- Serious long-term complications should be rare with high-quality surgery.

SUGGESTED CLINICAL STRATEGIES IN HAEMORRHOID MANAGEMENT

Grade I
Dietary and life-style changes. Add bulking agents if required.

Grade II
As above and consider banding. If treatment failure occurs, discuss surgery. Possible advantages of stapling.

Grade III
Unless patient unfit or strongly resistant to surgery then this should be advised. Should be given appropriate counselling regarding possibility of higher recurrence rates after stapling versus long-term complications of excisional procedures. Does anything require to be done to the external component? Excisional or stapling procedures both effective. If there is a substantial fixed external component requiring excision then advantages of stapling in better early pain control may be lost.

Grade IV
Surgery is the only reliably effective treatment. Balance of current evidence may favour excisional surgery; however, in appropriately experienced hands, stapled haemorrhoidopexy can produce very good results. Many patients will require some excision of a fixed external component.

PROLAPSED THROMBOSED HAEMORRHOIDS

Haemorrhoids may present with acute prolapse often as a result of massive straining or in pregnancy. This may rapidly progress to thrombosis or rarely gangrene. The condition is extremely painful but may generally be managed conservatively with analgesia, bulk laxatives, the topical application of heat and ice and a sphincter-relaxing agent. Surprisingly few patients subsequently require surgery for residual haemorrhoids. Historically, a minority of surgeons have carried out emergency surgery[35] but this seems to be associated with a high incidence of sphincter damage and subsequent continence problems. With the advent of stapling, some authors have reported satisfactory results for acute surgery.[36]

Key points for clinical practice

- Manual reduction of haemorrhoids is a strong indication for surgical treatment. Ask the patient if they manually reduce.

- The need for surgical treatment is largely driven by the effect of symptoms on quality of life.

- Important symptoms such as the need to reduce the haemorrhoids manually or soiling may not be readily volunteered.

- Flexible sigmoidoscopy is strongly recommended as a minimum in the investigation of patients with rectal bleeding.

(continued)

Key points for clinical practice *(continued)*

- Endo-anal ultrasound and anorectal physiology assessment is recommended in cases with a previous history suggesting obstetric trauma or iatrogenic injury.

- Metronidazole is the most important agent in reducing pain after haemorrhoid surgery.

- All forms of operative intervention have rarely been associated with serious complications.

- The presence of urinary difficulty associated with pelvic or lower abdominal pain and fever raises the problem of potentially life-threatening sepsis following haemorrhoid surgery.

- Patients can safely undergo day-case haemorrhoid surgery subject to the same medical and social criteria as for other procedures.

- Serious long-term complications should be rare with high-quality surgery.

References

1. Thomson WHF. The nature of haemorrhoids. *Br J Surg* 1975; **62**: 542–552.
2. Johanson JF, Sonnenberg A. Temporal changes in the occurrence of haemorrhoids in the United States and England. *Dis Colon Rectum* 1991; **34**: 585–591.
3. Alonso-Coello P, Mills E, Heels-Ansdell D, Lopez-Yarto M, Zhou Q, Johanson JF, Guyatt G. Fiber for the treatment of hemorrhoids complications: a systematic review and meta-analysis. *Am J Gastroenterol* 2006; **101**: 181–188.
4. Beattie GC, Wilson RG, Loudon MA. The contemporary management of haemorrhoids. *Colorect Dis* 2002; **4**: 450–454.
5. Watson NF, Liptrott S, Maxwell-Armstrong CA. A prospective audit of early pain and patient satisfaction following out-patient band ligation of haemorrhoids. *Ann R Coll Surg Engl* 2006; **88**: 275–279.
6. Shanmugam V, Thaha MA, Rabindranath KS, Campbell KL, Steele RJC, Loudon MA. Systematic review of randomized trials comparing rubber band ligation with excisional haemorrhoidectomy. *Br J Surg* 2005; **92**: 1481–1487.
7. Longman RJ, Thomson WH. A prospective study of outcome from rubber band ligation of piles. *Colorect Dis* 2006; **8**: 145–148.
8. Milligan ET, Morgan CN, Jones LE, Officer R. Surgical anatomy of the anal canal and the operative treatment of haemorrhoids. *Lancet* 1937; **ii**: 1119–1124.
9. Ferguson JA, Heaton JR. Closed haemorrhoidectomy. *Dis Colon Rectum* 1959; **2**: 176–179.
10. Carapeti EA, Kamm MA, McDonald PJ, Phillips RK. Double-blind randomised controlled trial of effect of metronidazole on pain after day-case haemorrhoidectomy. *Lancet* 1998; **351**: 169–172.
11. Ng S, Siu-Man L, Fung-Yee J et al. Pre-emptive analgesia and metronidazole on post-haemorrhoidectomy pain control. *Surg Pract* 2006; **10**: 102–105.
12. Silverman R, Bendick PJ, Wasvary HJ. A randomized, prospective, double-blind, placebo-controlled trial of the effect of a calcium channel blocker ointment on pain after hemorrhoidectomy. *Dis Colon Rectum* 2005; **48**: 1913–1916.
13. Johannsson HO, Pahlman L, Graf W. Randomized clinical trial of the effects on anal function of Milligan-Morgan versus Ferguson Haemorrhoidectomy. *Br J Surg* 2006; **93**: 1208–1114.

14. Longo A. Treatment of haemorrhoidal disease by reduction of mucosa and haemorrhoidal prolapse with a circular stapling device: a new procedure. *6th World Congress of Endoscopic Surgery*. Naples: Mundozzi, 1998; 777–784.

15. Corman ML, Gravie J-F, Hager T *et al*. Stapled haemorrhoidopexy: a consensus position paper by an international working party – indications, contra-indications and technique. *Colorect Dis* 2003; **5**: 304–310.

16. Ng KH, Ho KS, Ooi BS, Tang CL, Eu KW. Experience of 3711 stapled haemorrhoidectomy operations. *Br J Surg* 2006; **93**: 226–230.

17. Felice G, Privitera A, Ellul E, Klaumann M. Doppler-guided hemorrhoidal artery ligation: an alternative to hemorrhoidectomy. *Dis Colon Rectum* 2005; **48**: 2090–2093.

18. Greenberg R, Karin E, Avital S, Skornick Y, Werbin N. First 100 cases with Doppler-guided hemorrhoidal artery ligation. *Dis Colon Rectum* 2006; **49**: 485–489.

19. Ramirez JM, Gracia JA, Aguilella V, Elia M, Casamayor MC, Martinez M. Surgical management of symptomatic haemorrhoids: to cut, to hang or to strangle? A prospective randomized controlled trial. *Colorect Dis* 2005; **7 (Suppl. 2)**: 52.

20. Guenin MO, Rosenthal R, Kern B, Peterli R, von Flue M, Ackermann C. Ferguson hemorrhoidectomy: long-term results and patient satisfaction after Ferguson's hemorrhoidectomy. *Dis Colon Rectum* 2005; **48**: 1523–1527.

21. Justin TA, Armitage NC. Haemorrhoidectomy: 5 years later. *Br J Surg* 1999; **86 (Suppl. 1)**: 60.

22. Winter A, Sharp CM, Wright DM, Sunderland GT. Long-term outcome following daycase haemorrhoidectomy. *Colorect Dis* 2000; **2 (Suppl. 1)**: 67.

23. Sutherland LM, Burchard AK, Matsuda K *et al*. A systematic review of stapled haemorrhoidectomy. *Arch Surg* 2002; **137**: 1395–1406.

24. Beattie GC, Loudon MA. Follow-up confirms sustained benefit of circumferential stapled anoplasty in the management of prolapsing haemorrhoids. *Br J Surg* 2001; **88**: 850–852.

25. Shanmugam V, Loudon MA. Stapled haemorrhoidopexy is effective in long-term control of haemorrhoidal symptoms: 109 cases. *Colorect Dis* 2005; **7 (Suppl. 1)**: 37–38.

26. Bullock N. Impotence after sclerotherapy of haemorrhoids: case reports. *BMJ* 1997; **314**: 419.

27. Barwell J, Watkins RM, Lloyd-Davies E, Wilkins DC. Life-threatening retroperitoneal sepsis after hemorrhoid injection sclerotherapy: report of a case. *Dis Colon Rectum* 1999; **42**: 421–423.

28. Guy RJ, Seow-Choen F. Septic complications after treatment of haemorrhoids. *Br J Surg* 2003; **90**: 147–156.

29. Molloy RG, Kingsmore D. Life threatening pelvic sepsis after stapled haemorrhoidectomy. *Lancet* 2000; **355**: 810.

30. McCloud JM, Jameson JS, Scott AND. Life-threatening sepsis following treatment for haemorrhoids: a systematic review. *Colorect Dis* 2006; **8**: 748–755.

31. Carapeti EA, Kamm MA, McDonald PJ, Chadwick SJ, Phillips RK. Randomized trial of open versus closed day-case haemorrhoidectomy. *Br J Surg* 1999; **86**: 612–613.

32. Tjandra J. Ambulatory haemorrhoidectomy – has the time come? *Aust NZ J Surg* 2005; **75**: 183.

33. Beattie GC, McAdam TK, McIntosh SA, Loudon MA. Day case stapled haemorrhoidopexy for prolapsing haemorrhoids. *Colorect Dis* 2006; **8**: 56–61.

34. Thaha MA, Irvine LA, Steele RJ, Campbell KL. Postdefaecation pain syndrome after circular stapled anopexy is abolished by oral nifedipine. *Br J Surg* 2005; **92**: 208–210.

35. Allan A, Samad AJ, Mellon A, Marshall T. Prospective randomised study of urgent haemorrhoidectomy compared with non-operative treatment in the management of prolapsed thrombosed internal haemorrhoids. *Colorect Dis* 2006; **8**: 41–45.

36. Kang JC, Chung MH, Chao PC, Lee CC, Hsiao CW, Jao SW. Emergency stapled haemorrhoidectomy for haemorrhoidal crisis. *Br J Surg* 2005; **92**: 1014–1016.

Richard E. Lovegrove Paris P. Tekkis

11

Functional outcome following restorative proctocolectomy

Since the first description of restorative proctocolectomy in 1978 by Parks and Nicholls,[1] patients requiring proctocolectomy for ulcerative colitis and familial adenomatous polyposis may no longer face the prospect of life with a permanent ileostomy. The initial description was of a three-limbed S pouch and a hand-sewn pouch-anal anastomosis after mucosectomy of the anorectum. Over the years, a number of technical refinements were made, namely: (i) introduction of the two-limbed J[2] and four-limbed W[3] reservoir; and (ii) the use of surgical stapling devices for pouch construction and creation of the pouch-anal anastomosis.[4]

Restorative proctocolectomy is known to be associated with significant short- and long-term adverse events, with ileal pouch failure occurring in 10% of patients within 10 years of surgery. However, in those patients who retain the ileal pouch, functional outcomes are generally good. The assessment of functional outcome is made during routine follow-up, after reversal of the defunctioning ileostomy, where applicable. Stool frequency, faecal urgency, seepage of liquid matter from the pouch, incontinence to stool, and the need to wear protective pads are important markers of pouch function and may provide a subjective assessment of anal sphincter and reservoir function. Many patients require antidiarrhoeal medication in order to thicken the consistency of their stool, thus reducing stool frequency and the risk of seepage. Scoring systems to quantify overall pouch function have been described,[5] but these have not gained wide-spread acceptance in clinical use. Pouch function varies throughout the follow-up period, with occasional transient or persistent deterioration in function representing the onset of adverse events comprising

Richard E. Lovegrove MRCS (for correspondence)
Clinical Research Fellow, Imperial College London, ROOM 1003, 10th Floor QEQM Building, St Mary's Hospital, London W2 1NY, UK. rlovegrove@doctors.org.uk

Paris P. Tekkis MD FRCS
Senior Clinical Lecturer and Conslltant Colorectal Surgeon, Department of Biosurgery & Surgical Technology, Imperial College London and St Mary's Hospital, London, UK; and Honorary Consultant Colorectal Surgeon, Department of Colorectal Surgery, St Mark's Hospital, Harrow, UK

a wide host of differential diagnoses including: pouchitis;[6] pre-pouch obstructive ileitis or pouch ileitis; stricture at any level proximal to the pouch, within the pouch or at the pouch-anal anastomosis; peri-pouch sepsis or fistulation; inflammation of the retained rectum (in the case of stapled anastomoses); low volume reservoir; or sphincter dysfunction.

POUCH DESIGN AND OUTCOME

The three common types of reservoir in use have different characteristics in terms of functional outcomes. Although the use of a J pouch currently predominates in procedures being undertaken, this is largely a product of its simple stapled construction and reduced operative time. The number of limbs utilised in the construction of the ileal pouch is proportional to its subsequent volume,[7,8] and it can be deduced that this has a subsequent effect on stool frequency.

S POUCH

The original S pouch, as described by Parks and Nicholls,[1] had a long efferent limb which led to difficulties in emptying the reservoir. In one series,[9] 59% of patients having an S pouch were unable to empty the pouch spontaneously and needed to intubate the reservoir with a catheter. Subsequently, the design of the S pouch was modified through elimination of the efferent limb, to allow spontaneous evacuation.[10] Although little used at present, the S pouch may provide additional length where a J or W pouch would not reach the anorectal remnant following proctectomy; therefore, it still has a role. The S pouch is associated with a stool frequency that is intermediate to that of the J and W designs, and patients have a reduced need for antidiarrhoeal medication compared to those with a J reservoir.[8]

J POUCH

The J pouch has the smallest volume of the three reservoirs. In a series of 203 patients from New Zealand, Neily et al.[11] reported a 24-hour stool frequency for the J pouch of 5.4 ± 1.9 motions, with 1.0 ± 0.6 of these occurring at night. This finding has been mirrored in the results of other investigators.[9,12] One study assessed whether increasing the length of small bowel used to fashion the J pouch from 30 cm to 40 cm would have any effect on functional outcomes.[13] The authors concluded that there was no significant advantage in pouch function when 40 cm of small bowel was used. The need for antidiarrhoeal medication has been reported with great variation in the literature, with between 23%[14] and 86%[15] of patients requiring these in order reduce their stool frequency.

W POUCH

The W pouch, comprising four limbs of ileum has a larger volume than either the J or S designs; consequently, it is associated with a decreased frequency of defecation.[9,16] In one study, it was found that 19 of 41 patients having a W

Table 1 Impact of factors on stool frequency following restorative proctocolectomy

		WMD	95% CI	P-value
24-hour stool frequency				
Pouch design[8]				
	S vs W	1.14	−0.10, 2.38	0.07
	S vs J	−1.48	−2.10, −0.85	< 0.01
	J vs W	0.97	0.20, 1.74	0.01
Diagnosis				
	UC vs FAP[35]	0.99	0.21, 1.76	0.01
	CD vs UC[36]	0.21	−0.46, 0.88	0.54
	CD vs IC[36]	0.70	−0.25, 1.66	0.15
Nocturnal stool frequency				
Pouch design[8]				
	S vs W	0.13	−0.06, 0.32	0.19
	S vs J	−0.06	−0.28, 0.15	0.55
	J vs W	0.21	−0.14, 0.56	0.25
Diagnosis				
	UC vs FAP[35]	0	−0.34, 0.34	1.00

WMD, weighted mean difference (difference in mean stool frequency between the two groups [a vs b, where WMD = mean(b) − mean(a)]).
UC, ulcerative colitis; IC, indeterminate colitis; CD, Crohn's disease; FAP, familial adenomatous polyposis; CI, confidence interval.

pouch were unable to empty their pouch spontaneously.[17] However, this finding has not been mirrored by other studies. Similarly, the need for antidiarrhoeal medication is reduced, particularly when compared to the J pouch.[17,18] The W pouch, however, is both technically demanding and time consuming to construct with the reservoir requiring hand-sewn anastomoses owing to its complexity.

Although several studies and a recent meta-analysis have shown statistically significant differences in 24-hour stool frequency, these amounted to 1–1.5 motions per 24 hours (Table 1), which is unlikely to be of any clinical significance. The incidence of incontinence, seepage, urgency and perineal excoriation were similar between the three reservoir designs (Tables 2 and 3). With its simpler, quicker construction and little difference in clinical functional outcome, it may be easy to see why the use of a J pouch has become the procedure of choice for many surgeons undertaking restorative proctocolectomy.

Key point 3

- Pouch volume increases with the number of limbs employed in its construction, with reduction in 24-hour stool frequencies.

HAND-SEWN VERSUS STAPLED POUCH-ANAL ANASTOMOSIS

In the original description of the ileal pouch by Parks and Nicholls,[1] the pouch-anal anastomosis was performed following a mucosectomy of the anal canal at the level of the dentate line and a hand-sewn anastomosis fashioned to the

Table 2 Factors affecting continence

	OR	95% CI	P-value
Seepage (day)			
Anastomosis[25]			
Hand-sewn vs stapled	1.94	0.84, 4.49	0.12
Diagnosis			
UC vs FAP[35]	0.84	0.24, 2.90	0.78
Pouch type[8]			
S vs W	3.01	0.80, 11.42	0.10
S vs J	0.83	0.34, 2.07	0.69
J vs W	2.42	0.70, 8.36	0.16
Seepage (night)			
Anastomosis[25]			
Hand-sewn vs stapled	2.78	1.70, 4.56	< 0.01
Diagnosis			
UC vs FAP[35]	1.02	0.26, 3.92	0.98
Pouch type[8]			
S vs W	2.67	0.60, 11.76	0.20
S vs J	0.60	0.16, 2.20	0.44
J vs W	1.56	0.46, 5.30	0.47
Incontinence			
Anastomosis[25]			
Hand-sewn vs stapled	2.32	1.24, 4.34	0.01
Diagnosis			
UC vs FAP[35]	0.28	0.05, 1.42	0.12
CD vs UC[36]	3.00	1.48, 6.08	< 0.01
CD vs IC[36]	2.25	0.68, 7.46	0.19
Pouch type[8]			
S vs W	1.02	0.26, 3.97	0.98
S vs J	0.95	0.29, 3.14	0.93
J vs W	2.31	0.34, 15.72	0.39

OR, odds ratio (risk of event in group a relative to group b [a vs b]).
UC, ulcerative colitis; IC, indeterminate colitis; CD, Crohn's disease; FAP, familial adenomatous polyposis; CI, confidence interval.

anoderm. This technique, although technically demanding and time consuming, is still widely in use as it has the advantage of removing most of the anal mucosa, therefore reducing the incidence of cuffitis which can often lead to functional impairment of the ileal pouch reservoir. During the early 1980s, as the use of surgical staplers gained popularity their use was turned to restorative proctocolectomy, and a number of authors have reported good functional results.[4] Proponents of a stapled technique would argue that the procedure is quicker to perform with less trauma to the anal sphincter complex, resulting in improved resting and squeeze pressures postoperatively.[19,20] Conversely, the undertaking of a hand-sewn anastomosis allows for excision of the diseased mucosa, thereby reducing the risk of polyp formation or inflammation in the retained rectal cuff. However, small islands of mucosa may remain, thereby not totally eliminating this risk.[21]

A number of studies have sought to compare functional outcomes between patients undergoing restorative proctocolectomy with a hand-sewn or stapled pouch-anal anastomosis,[22-24] and these have been recently pooled in a quantitative meta-analysis of 21 such studies.[25] It has been shown that the undertaking of a hand-sewn pouch-anal anastomosis was associated with significant reductions in the mean resting and squeeze pressure of 13.4 mmHg and 14.4 mmHg, respectively. This was associated with a trend towards increased seepage of stool during the day and a significant increase in the incidence of stool seepage at night in those patients having a hand-sewn anastomosis (Table 2). Similarly, episodes of frank incontinence were also increased in those patients undergoing hand-sewn anastomoses. Stool frequency over 24 hours and at night was not affected by the type of anastomosis, nor was the need for antidiarrhoeal medication (Table 1). None of the studies, however, have reported whether the apparent functional impairment seen in the hand-sewn ileal pouch group was a transient or permanent phenomenon. In clinical practice, it is likely that continence improves within the first 6 months of pouch formation and offsets some the adverse symptoms encountered once the intestinal continuity is restored.

Key point 1 & 2

- With the exception of Crohn's disease, the pre-operative diagnosis has little effect on stool frequency.

- Patients with Crohn's disease who inadvertently underwent restorative proctocolectomy, often experience significantly more urgency, faecal incontinence and, ultimately, ileal pouch failure.

The benefit of a stapled anastomosis in improved continence may, however, be offset by the development of inflammation of the retained rectal stump (cuffitis) which can lead to increased frequency, pain and urgency as seen in episodes of acute pouchitis. Patients undergoing a hand-sewn anastomosis have a 62% decreased risk of developing inflammation within the retained rectum[25] thus reducing the need for medical intervention.

It has been suggested[21] that patients with established colon or rectal cancer at the time of restorative proctocolectomy or having dysplasia in the distal two-thirds of the rectum should undergo a hand-sewn anastomosis in order to minimise the risk of neoplastic transformation within the retained rectal cuff. The authors feel that this is a justifiable approach, providing a balance between functional outcome and future risk, which is likely to necessitate further surgery. In addition, patients with severe distal proctitis should be considered for a hand-sewn anastomosis in order to decrease the risk of inflammation within the retained rectum.

Key point 4

- The undertaking of a hand-sewn anastomosis decreases anal sphincter pressure with consequent impairment of anal continence. It is of benefit in reducing the risk of inflammation and possibly neoplastic transformation in the rectal stump.

SELECTIVE OMISSION OF ILEOSTOMY

Restorative proctocolectomy without a covering loop ileostomy is one of the more controversial variations in the operative technique. Since the first published series by Everett et al.,[26] selective omission of an ileostomy has gained a number of proponents with generally acceptable results.[27,28] Arguments for inclusion of a loop ileostomy as part of the operative technique include diversion of the faecal stream away from the pouch-anal anastomosis, thereby minimising the risk of sepsis from an anastomotic leak and the psychological benefit to the patient of having lived with an ileostomy should their pouch subsequently fail. However, closure of the ileostomy was often associated with a complication rate of 11.4%,[29] an increased risk of pouch-anal anastomotic stricture[30] and, possibly, small bowel obstruction[31] in those patients having a covering ileostomy.

Following restorative proctocolectomy without a covering ileostomy there was a non-significant decrease in 24-hour stool frequency of 0.5 motions.[30] This may represent earlier restoration of ileal pouch compliance since the faecal stream enters the reservoir much sooner after surgery and facilitates expansion of the pouch. Similarly, an ileal pouch that has been defunctioned following restorative proctocolectomy would collapse down onto itself and may become less compliant. At the same time, the pouch-anal anastomosis often develops an asymptomatic stricture which requires regular digitation at 4–6-weekly intervals to prevent irreversible symptomatic stricturing. These can lead to early pouch dysfunction with increased stool frequency following reversal of the ileostomy. Continence and the need for antidiarrhoeal medication did not differ in those patients operated on with or without a covering ileostomy. Other studies have found no significant differences in functional outcomes between these groups.[32]

Following closure of a covering loop ileostomy, small bowel obstruction has been reported to occur in 6.4% of patients. In a series of 1504 patients having ileostomy reversal following restorative proctocolectomy, it was found that 1 patient (0.07%) had developed an anastomotic stricture at the closure site.[29] Whilst the risk of stricture at the closure site was small, in the ileal pouch patient this may manifest itself as increased stool frequency with associated urgency. In patients where pouch function is not improving following ileostomy closure, a contrast study is often useful to exclude the presence of such a stricture.

Key point 5

- Selective omission of a loop ileostomy has no long-term effect on functional outcomes following restorative proctocolectomy although patients should be warned of a difficult early postoperative recovery.

EFFECT OF UNDERLYING DIAGNOSIS

Restorative proctocolectomy is primarily undertaken in patients with familial adenomatous polyposis or ulcerative colitis. However, some authors believe that isolated colonic Crohn's disease should remain an indication for restorative proctocolectomy.[33] While familial adenomatous polyposis or ulcerative colitis are principally diseases of the colonic mucosa, Crohn's disease can affect any part of the gastrointestinal tract and is associated with transmural inflammation. A diagnosis of indeterminate colitis may be made in some patients where the pathological features of Crohn's disease or ulcerative colitis are unclear. Under these circumstances, many surgeons would proceed with restorative proctocolectomy, but would undertake this as a staged procedure to allow the pathologist to review the colectomy specimen in the hope that, by providing the pathologist with a large amount of tissue, a diagnosis of ulcerative colitis or Crohn's disease can be reached.

Patients with ulcerative colitis experience episodes of frequency and urgency during acute attacks of colitis. In many cases, the urgency experienced can be incapacitating and may prompt the patient to seek out surgical options. In contrast, patients with familial adenomatous polyposis have relatively normal bowel function prior to surgical intervention. A proportion of patients with familial adenomatous polyposis undergo total colectomy with ileorectal anastomosis prior to the restorative proctocolectomy. Whilst an ileorectal anastomosis is associated with decreased stool frequency compared to restorative proctocolectomy, reported urgency may be greater.[34]

A number of studies exist comparing outcomes following restorative proctocolectomy between these diagnoses.[35–38] Whilst some authors have shown greatly reduced 24-hour and nocturnal stool frequency in patients with familial adenomatous polyposis,[39] it is more likely that these differences are much smaller, amounting to one extra motion per 24 hours in patients with ulcerative colitis, and no difference in the overnight stool frequency (Table 1).[35] In those patients operated on with a diagnosis of Crohn's disease, there does not appear to be a significant difference in stool frequency when compared to patients with ulcerative colitis or indeterminate colitis.[36] However, patients undergoing restorative proctocolectomy for Crohn's disease were more likely to experience urgency and incontinence than patients with ulcerative colitis (Table 3). Episodes of urgency and incontinence did not differ significantly between patients with ulcerative colitis and familial adenomatous polyposis during follow-up.

Table 3 Factors affecting urgency

	OR	95% CI	P-value
Diagnosis			
UC vs FAP[35]	1.76	0.57, 5.42	0.32
CD vs UC[36]	2.75	1.02, 7.37	0.04
CD vs IC[36]	1.65	0.61, 4.46	0.32
Pouch type[8]			
S vs W	2.63	0.47, 14.74	0.27
S vs J	0.59	0.23, 1.54	0.28
J vs W	1.35	0.47, 3.92	0.58

OR, odds ratio (risk of event in group a relative to group b [a vs b]).
UC, ulcerative colitis; IC, indeterminate colitis; CD, Crohn's disease; FAP, familial adenomatous polyposis; CI, confidence interval.

Pouchitis is the development of inflammation within the ileal pouch and may be associated with increased stool frequency, incontinence, the passage of blood *per rectum*, fever and abdominal pain. The exact aetiology remains unknown, but it is seen predominantly in patients who underwent restorative proctocolectomy for ulcerative colitis. The majority of patients are diagnosed as having pouchitis based on clinical or endoscopic criteria. However, by performing pouchoscopy, it is possible to visualise areas of inflammation and take biopsies to confirm the diagnosis based on histological criteria. Patients with ulcerative colitis are 6.4 times more likely to develop pouchitis than patients with familial adenomatous polyposis when all assessment criteria are considered, rising to 17 times more likely if the diagnosis is made histologically.[35] Patients with Crohn's disease show a trend towards increased incidence of pouchitis when compared to either ulcerative colitis or indeterminate colitis.[36] If patients are experiencing repeated episodes of pouchitis, then this will have significant implications on their overall functional outcome and quality of life. In severe cases of chronic antibiotic-resistance pouchitis, patients may request to have their pouch defunctioned or excised.

POUCH FUNCTION WITH TIME

Following restorative proctocolectomy or reversal of the covering ileostomy, where applicable, many patients experience urgency, seepage and relatively high stool frequency. This steadily improves over the first 6 months, with further, smaller, improvements thereafter. During this period, the pouch is expanding and compliance is improving. The anal sphincters are recovering from the trauma of surgery, leading to improved continence. In those patients in whom a hand-sewn anastomosis has been fashioned, there may have been injury to the rich sensory supply in the anal transition zone with alteration in the ability to discriminate between stool and flatus.[40,41] As the pouch begins to function following ileostomy reversal, a process of 're-learning' occurs in the discriminatory ability of the anorectum and subsequent improvement in continence.

A large, multicentre study from the UK reported on functional outcomes following restorative proctocolectomy in 2491 patients, with maximum follow-up of 28 years.[42] Stool frequency over 24 hours demonstrated gradual improvement over the follow-up period, with a median of 5 motions per 24 hours at more than 20 years' follow-up. Whilst seepage of stool demonstrated improvement between 1–3 years' follow-up, thereafter there was steady deterioration in continence with the incidence of seepage rising from 3.9% to 20.5% during the day and 8.0% to 15.4% at night beyond 20 years' follow-up.

Another study from the University of Chicago,[43] with follow-up over 10 years, found that the number of motions per 24 hours decreased with increasing follow-up, whilst nocturnal frequency remained steady at 1 motion per night. Furthermore, the authors reported that the need for antimotility drugs decreased, whilst the use of fibre preparations increased over the follow-up period.

Most patients can be re-assured that following restorative proctocolectomy their stool frequency will steadily improve with improvements in continence and urgency. However, as the follow-up period lengthens, together with ageing of the patient and associated alterations in anal sphincter physiology, there may be deterioration in continence and greater need for bulking agents or antimotility drugs.

> ## Key point 6
> - Stool frequency and urgency improve with duration of follow-up, but continence deteriorates following 15 years' follow-up.

MANAGEMENT OF POUCH DYSFUNCTION

While the majority of patients are able to maintain good pouch function with median 24-hour stool frequency of 4–6 motions, some patients may experience reservoir dysfunction. The causes for this are varied and the more common ones are summarised in Table 4.

Pouchitis is characterised by an increase in 24-hour stool frequency of more than 2 motions above normal for that patient, the onset of fever, stool consistency becoming liquid and the development of faecal urgency. Up to 30% of all patients undergoing restorative proctocolectomy develop pouchitis, with those having a pouch for ulcerative colitis being at greatest risk. If pouchoscopy is undertaken there may be focal areas of inflammation or ulceration, or the appearance of this may be more confluent. Biopsies can be taken to allow more accurate severity assessment and help to differentiate between acute and chronic inflammation. Pouchitis can be treated with antibiotics, of which ciprofloxacin or metronidazole either in monotherapy or combined can be used. Initially, a 1-week course in high dose should be tried,

Table 4 The effect of complications on functional outcomes

Complication	Functional manifestation	Other manifestations	Investigation
Pouchitis	Liquid stool, blood, urgency	Abdominal pain, fever	Pouchoscopy and biopsy
Chronic intestinal obstruction	Liquid stool	Abdominal pain and distension	Plain or contrast radiology, CT
Evacuation disorders			
Ileoanal stenosis	Frequent, small volume stool		Digital examination, pouchogram
Long distal segment	Frequent, small volume stool. May need to intubate		Pouchogram
'Functional'			
Low capacitance reservoir	Frequent, small volume stool. Urgency		Pouchogram
'Functional' frequency	Phasic frequency		Ambulant pressure monitoring

followed by a 2–4 week course in low dose should this fail. A small number of patients developing pouchitis will go on to have many acute episodes (acute-relapsing pouchitis) or develop chronic pouchitis. In these patients, the administration of probiotics may help quiesce symptoms.

Key point 7

- Dysfunction of the ileal pouch may represent the onset of a new complication and should be investigated fully.

Obstructive symptoms occur at three principal levels: (i) the site of ileostomy closure; (ii) the afferent limb to the pouch; or (iii) at the ileoanal anastomosis. When obstructive symptoms are present, the pouch-anal anastomosis should be digitated to assess the efferent lumen. Stenosis of the pouch-anal anastomosis occurs in up to 30% of patients, and is more likely in those patients who were defunctioned at the time of surgery. A sigmoidoscope can then be passed into the pouch, and the pouch inlet can be visualised. Using a flexible sigmoidoscope, it may be possible to pass the scope through the afferent limb to the level of the ileostomy closure to assess for stenosis at this level. If this is not possible, a contrast study can be obtained to assess for evidence of obstruction. A stricture of the pouch-anal anastomosis can be treated through the use of anal dilators or, more rarely, surgical dilatation if the stricture is fibrotic. More proximal obstruction may require laparotomy in order to resolve it.

A long distal segment, as seen in the early S reservoirs, may cause difficulty in evacuation of the pouch. Patients may be happy to intubate the pouch since this provides them with control over when to evacuate and may be preferable to a high frequency if this were not the case. In those patients who cannot tolerate intubation, the reservoir may need to be refashioned to eliminate the distal segment.

A low capacitance reservoir will fill more quickly than larger reservoirs, resulting in increased stool frequency and urgency. The three and four limb S and W reservoirs are more spherical than the two limb J and achieve greater intraluminal volumes. The reservoir may also become contracted as a result of persistent pouchitis or persistent peri-pouch sepsis. The capacity of the reservoir can be assessed from pouchography or balloon volumetry. Patients should be given antidiarrhoeal medication in an attempt to control frequency. If unacceptable frequency persists, the patient may be offered a revision of the reservoir or to have the pouch defunctioned or excised.

Key points for clinical practice

- With the exception of Crohn's disease, the pre-operative diagnosis has little effect on stool frequency.

- Patients with Crohn's disease who inadvertently underwent restorative proctocolectomy, often experience significantly more urgency, faecal incontinence and, ultimately, ileal pouch failure.

(continued)

Key points for clinical practice *(continued)*

- Pouch volume increases with the number of limbs employed in its construction, with reduction in 24-hour stool frequencies.

- The undertaking of a hand-sewn anastomosis decreases anal sphincter pressure with consequent impairment of anal continence. It is of benefit in reducing the risk of inflammation and possibly neoplastic transformation in the rectal stump.

- Selective omission of a loop ileostomy has no long-term effect on functional outcomes following restorative proctocolectomy although patients should be warned of a difficult early postoperative recovery.

- Stool frequency and urgency improve with duration of follow-up, but continence deteriorates following 15 years' follow-up.

- Dysfunction of the ileal pouch may represent the onset of a new complication and should be investigated fully..

References

1. Parks AG, Nicholls RJ. Proctocolectomy without ileostomy for ulcerative colitis. *BMJ* 1978; **2**: 85–88.
2. Utsunomiya J, Iwama T, Imajo M *et al*. Total colectomy, mucosal proctectomy, and ileoanal anastomosis. *Dis Colon Rectum* 1980; **23**: 459–466.
3. Nicholls RJ, Lubowski DZ. Restorative proctocolectomy: the four loop (W) reservoir. *Br J Surg* 1987; **74**: 564–566.
4. Kmiot WA, Keighley MR. Totally stapled abdominal restorative proctocolectomy. *Br J Surg* 1989; **76**: 961–964.
5. Deen KI, Williams JG, Grant EA *et al*. Randomized trial to determine the optimum level of pouch-anal anastomosis in stapled restorative proctocolectomy. *Dis Colon Rectum* 1995; **38**: 133–138.
6. Hurst RD, Chung TP, Rubin M, Michelassi F. The implications of acute pouchitis on the long-term functional results after restorative proctocolectomy. *Inflamm Bowel Dis* 1998; **4**: 280–284.
7. Hallgren T, Fasth S, Nordgren S *et al*. Manovolumetric characteristics and functional results in three different pelvic pouch designs. *Int J Colorect Dis* 1989; **4**: 156–160.
8. Lovegrove RE, Heriot AG, Constantinides VA *et al*. A comparison of short-term and long-term outcomes of J, W and S ileal pouch reservoirs for restorative proctocolectomy. *Colorect Dis* 2006; DOI 10.1111/j.1463–1318.2006.01093.x
9. Nicholls RJ, Pezim ME. Restorative proctocolectomy with ileal reservoir for ulcerative colitis and familial adenomatous polyposis: a comparison of three reservoir designs. *Br J Surg* 1985; **72**: 470–474.
10. Pescatori M. A modified three-loop ileoanal reservoir. *Dis Colon Rectum* 1988; **31**: 823–824.
11. Neilly P, Neill ME, Hill GL. Restorative proctocolectomy with ileal pouch-anal anastomosis in 203 patients: the Auckland experience. *Aust NZ J Surg* 1999; **69**: 22–27.
12. Selvaggi F, Giuliani A, Gallo C *et al*. Randomized, controlled trial to compare the J-pouch and W-pouch configurations for ulcerative colitis in the maturation period. *Dis Colon Rectum* 2000; **43**: 615–620.
13. Johnston D, Williamson ME, Lewis WG *et al*. Prospective controlled trial of duplicated (J) versus quadruplicated (W) pelvic ileal reservoirs in restorative proctocolectomy for ulcerative colitis. *Gut* 1996; **39**: 242–247.
14. Schoetz Jr DJ, Coller JA, Veidenheimer MC. Ileoanal reservoir for ulcerative colitis and familial polyposis. *Arch Surg* 1986; **121**: 404–409.

15. Nasmyth DG, Williams NS, Johnston D. Comparison of the function of triplicated and duplicated pelvic ileal reservoirs after mucosal proctectomy and ileo-anal anastomosis for ulcerative colitis and adenomatous polyposis. *Br J Surg* 1986; **73**: 361–366.
16. Harms BA, Pahl AC, Starling JR. Comparison of clinical and compliance characteristics between S and W ileal reservoirs. *Am J Surg* 1990; **159**: 34–39.
17. Romanos J, Samarasekera DN, Stebbing JF *et al*. Outcome of 200 restorative proctocolectomy operations: the John Radcliffe Hospital experience. *Br J Surg* 1997; **84**: 814–818.
18. de Silva HJ, de Angelis CP, Soper N *et al*. Clinical and functional outcome after restorative proctocolectomy. *Br J Surg* 1991; **78**: 1039–1044.
19. Reilly WT, Pemberton JH, Wolff BG *et al*. Randomized prospective trial comparing ileal pouch-anal anastomosis performed by excising the anal mucosa to ileal pouch-anal anastomosis performed by preserving the anal mucosa. *Ann Surg* 1997; **225**: 666–676.
20. Saigusa N, Kurahashi T, Nakamura T *et al*. Functional outcome of stapled ileal pouch-anal canal anastomosis versus handsewn pouch-anal anastomosis. *Surg Today* 2000; **30**: 575–581.
21. Remzi FH, Fazio VW, Delaney CP *et al*. Dysplasia of the anal transitional zone after ileal pouch-anal anastomosis: results of prospective evaluation after a minimum of ten years. *Dis Colon Rectum* 2003; **46**: 6–13.
22. Gemlo BT, Belmonte C, Wiltz O, Madoff RD. Functional assessment of ileal pouch-anal anastomotic techniques. *Am J Surg* 1995; **169**: 137–141.
23. Gozzetti G, Poggioli G, Marchetti F *et al*. Functional outcome in handsewn versus stapled ileal pouch-anal anastomosis. *Am J Surg* 1994; **168**: 325–329.
24. Remzi FH, Church JM, Bast J *et al*. Mucosectomy vs. stapled ileal pouch-anal anastomosis in patients with familial adenomatous polyposis: functional outcome and neoplasia control. *Dis Colon Rectum* 2001; **44**: 1590–1596.
25. Lovegrove RE, Constantinides VA, Heriot AG *et al*. A Comparison of hand-sewn versus stapled ileal pouch anal anastomosis (IPAA) following proctocolectomy: a meta-analysis of 4183 patients. *Ann Surg* 2006; **244**: 18–26.
26. Everett WG, Pollard SG. Restorative proctocolectomy without temporary ileostomy. *Br J Surg* 1990; **77**: 621–622.
27. Gorfine SR, Gelernt IM, Bauer JJ *et al*. Restorative proctocolectomy without diverting ileostomy. *Dis Colon Rectum* 1995; **38**: 188–194.
28. Grobler SP, Hosie KB, Keighley MR. Randomized trial of loop ileostomy in restorative proctocolectomy. *Br J Surg* 1992; **79**: 903–906.
29. Wong KS, Remzi FH, Gorgun E *et al*. Loop ileostomy closure after restorative proctocolectomy: outcome in 1,504 patients. *Dis Colon Rectum* 2005; **48**: 243–250.
30. Weston-Petrides GK, Lovegrove RE, Tilney HS *et al*. Comparison of outcomes following restorative proctocolectomy with or without defunctioning ileostomy. *Arch Surg* 2006; In press.
31. Remzi FH, Fazio VW, Gorgun E *et al*. The outcome after restorative proctocolectomy with or without defunctioning ileostomy. *Dis Colon Rectum* 2006; **49**: 470–477.
32. Mowschenson PM, Critchlow JF, Peppercorn MA. Ileoanal pouch operation: long-term outcome with or without diverting ileostomy. *Arch Surg* 2000; **135**: 463–465.
33. Panis Y. Is there a place for ileal pouch-anal anastomosis in patients with Crohn's colitis? *Neth J Med* 1998; **53**: S47–S51.
34. Aziz O, Athanasiou T, Fazio VW *et al*. Meta-analysis of observational studies of ileorectal versus ileal pouch-anal anastomosis for familial adenomatous polyposis. *Br J Surg* 2006; **93**: 407–417.
35. Lovegrove RE, Tilney HS, Heriot AG *et al*. A comparison of adverse events and functional outcomes after restorative proctocolectomy for familial adenomatous polyposis and ulcerative colitis. *Dis Colon Rectum* 2006; **49**: 1293–1306.
36. Reese GE, Lovegrove RE, Tilney HS *et al*. The effect of Crohn's disease on outcomes following restorative proctocolectomy. *Dis Colon Rectum* 2006; DOI 10.1007/s10350–006–0777–x
37. Regimbeau JM, Panis Y, Pocard M *et al*. Long-term results of ileal pouch-anal anastomosis for colorectal Crohn's disease. *Dis Colon Rectum* 2001; **44**: 769–778.
38. Tjandra JJ, Fazio VW, Church JM *et al*. Similar functional results after restorative proctocolectomy in patients with familial adenomatous polyposis and mucosal

ulcerative colitis. *Am J Surg* 1993; **165**: 322–325.

39. Braun J, Treutner KH, Schumpelick V. Stapled ileal pouch-anal anastomosis with resection of the anal transition zone. *Int J Colorect Dis* 1995; **10**: 142–147.

40. Duthie HL, Gairns FW. Sensory nerve-endings and sensation in the anal region of man. *Br J Surg* 1960; **47**: 585–595.

41. Miller R, Lewis GT, Bartolo DC *et al.* Sensory discrimination and dynamic activity in the anorectum: evidence using a new ambulatory technique. *Br J Surg* 1988; **75**: 1003–1007.

42. Tekkis PP. *A report on the National Ileal Pouch Registry.* Gateshead, UK: The Association of Coloproctology of Great Britain and Ireland. 2006.

43. Michelassi F, Lee J, Rubin M *et al.* Long-term functional results after ileal pouch anal restorative proctocolectomy for ulcerative colitis: a prospective observational study. *Ann Surg* 2003; **238**: 433–441.

Sayed Aly Clom J. Power Stephen G.E. Barker

12

Intestinal ischaemia

Occlusion of the mesenteric vessels is apt to be regarded as one of those conditions of which the diagnosis is impossible, the prognosis hopeless, and the treatment almost useless.

Cokkinis A.J. 1926[1]

Occlusive mesenteric ischaemia can be divided into acute and chronic forms: Acute mesenteric ischaemia (AMI) is a syndrome in which sudden, inadequate blood flow through the mesenteric circulation causes ischaemia and eventually, gangrene of the bowel wall. It can be arterial, or venous in aetiology. It has an in-hospital mortality rate of 59–93%.[2]

Chronic mesenteric ischaemia (CMI) and its associated 'abdominal angina', arises from long-standing, subacute, inadequate blood flow and is unlikely to develop unless significant stenoses (or occlusions) affect at least two of the following – coeliac artery, superior mesenteric artery, or inferior mesenteric artery. This form of ischaemia has an excellent prognosis, with low operative mortality and long-term survival rates of 50–60%.[3]

Key point 1

- Acute mesenteric ischaemia has an in-hospital mortality rate of 59–93% while chronic mesenteric ischaemia has an excellent prognosis, with low operative mortality and long-term survival rates of 50–60%.

Sayed Aly PhD FRCS (for correspondence)
Consultant Vascular and Endovascular Surgeon, Mater University Hospital, Dublin 7, Ireland
E-mail: sayed@doctors.org.uk

Clom J. Power MD FRCS
SpR in Surgery, Mater University Hospital, Dublin 7, Ireland

Stephen G.E. Barker MS FRCS
Senior Lecturer in Surgery, University College London, Gower Street, London W1, UK

ANATOMICAL CONSIDERATIONS

The bowels are supplied with three blood vessels. The coeliac axis divides into the left gastric artery, common hepatic artery and splenic mesenteric artery (SMA). These arteries provide blood to the stomach, duodenum, pancreas and liver. A rich collateral circulation exists (via pancreaticoduodenal arcades) between the coeliac axis and the SMA, accounting for the rarity of ischaemic events affecting these organs.

The SMA gives rise to the inferior pancreaticoduodenal artery, middle colic artery, right colic artery, and ileocolic artery. Bowel is perfused through a series of arterial arcades, supplying a terminal arcade which gives rise to multiple

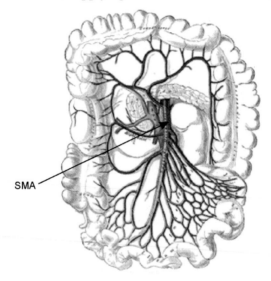

Fig. 1 Splenic mesenteric artery (SMA) and its branches.

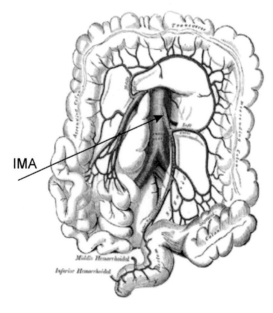

Fig. 2 Inferior mesenteric artery (IMA) and its branches.

straight-end arteries directly supplying the intestinal wall. The absence of collateral pathways at this level renders the small intestine particularly vulnerable to ischaemic events.

This design 'weakness' is offset by a collateral circulation between the SMA and inferior mesenteric artery (IMA) – the marginal artery of Drummond. Furthermore, the internal iliac arteries may provide collateral hindgut and midgut perfusion in the presence of an IMA occlusion (Figs 1 and 2)

Venous intestinal drainage consists mainly of the portal vein, which is the combination of SMV and splenic vein. IMV ends in the splenic vein.

PATHOPHYSIOLOGICAL CONSIDERATIONS

Damage to the bowel portion affected can range from reversible ischaemia to trans-mural infarction with necrosis and perforation. The injury is complicated by reactive vasospasm in the SMA region after the initial occlusion. Arterial insufficiency causes tissue hypoxia, leading to early bowel wall spasm. This tends to promote gut emptying with vomiting and/or diarrhoea. Mucosal sloughing may cause bleeding into the gastrointestinal tract. Usually, at this stage, little abdominal tenderness is present, resulting in the classic 'intense visceral pain disproportionate to physical examination findings'.

The mucosal barrier becomes disrupted as the ischaemia persists and bacteria, toxins, and vasoactive substances are released into the systemic circulation. This can cause death from septic shock, cardiac failure, or multisystem organ failure before bowel necrosis actually occurs. As hypoxic damage worsens, the bowel wall becomes oedematous and appears cyanotic. Fluid is released into the peritoneal cavity, explaining the presence of sero-sanguinous fluid sometimes recovered following diagnostic peritoneal lavage. Bowel necrosis occurs in 8–12 hours from the onset of symptoms. Transmural necrosis leads to peritoneal signs and heralds a much worse prognosis.

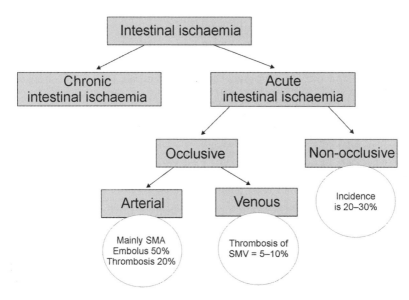

Fig. 3. Classification of intestinal ischaemia.

ACUTE MESENTERIC ISCHAEMIA (AMI)

Four primary clinical entities are known (Fig. 3): (i) acute mesenteric arterial embolus (AMAE); (ii) acute mesenteric arterial thrombosis (AMAT); (iii) non-occlusive mesenteric ischaemia (NOMI); and (iv) mesenteric venous thrombosis (MVT).

Acute mesenteric arterial embolus (AMAE)

The SMA is the visceral vessel most susceptible to emboli because of its acute take-off angle from the aorta and its relatively higher basal flow rate, accounting for > 50% of cases of AMI. Some 15% of the emboli remain impacted at the origin of the vessel. Most often, however, emboli lodge about 5–10 cm beyond the arterial origin, at a narrowing near the emergence of the middle colic artery.

Typical causes of embolisation include: mural thrombi after myocardial infarction, atrial thrombi associated with mitral stenosis and atrial fibrillation, vegetative endocarditis, mycotic aneurysm, and thrombi which form at the site of atheromatous plaques within the aorta, or at the sites of vascular aortic prosthetic grafts interposed between the heart and the origin of the SMA. Emboli can be of malignant origin (for example, atrial myxoma, or renal cell carcinoma), or be cholesterol emboli associated with diagnostic, or interventional, arteriographic catheter manipulation.

Whatever the aetiology, the vascular occlusion is sudden and patients are unable to develop a compensatory increase in collateral flow. As a result, they tend to experience worse ischaemia than patients with thrombotic AMI.

Acute mesenteric arterial thrombosis (AMAT)

This group accounts for about 20% of cases of AMI and is due to thrombosis on top of a pre-existing atherosclerotic lesion, within a visceral artery.

Most patients are female and have symptomatic, systemic vascular disease. Frequently, they have intestinal angina before the emergent event and, often, have undergone previous vascular surgery. Symptoms do not develop until two of the three arteries are stenosed, or completely blocked. Progressive worsening of the atherosclerotic stenosis before the acute occlusion often allows time for the development of an additional collateral circulation. Thrombotic AMI may be a complication of arterial aneurysm, or other vascular pathologies such as dissection trauma, and thromboangitis obliterans. In inflammatory vascular disease, smaller vessels are affected. Thrombosis tends to occur at the origin of the SMA causing wide-spread infarction.

Non-occlusive mesenteric ischaemia (NOMI)

This is responsible for between 20–30% of AMI (Fig. 4). It has been defined both as mesenteric vasoconstriction following gut hypoperfusion, or intestinal necrosis with a patent arterial tree. It is the most lethal form of AMI, with mortality rates of 70–100%. NOMI is precipitated by a severe reduction in mesenteric perfusion, with secondary arterial spasm, from such causes as cardiac failure, septic shock, hypovolaemia, or the use of potent vasopressors in patients in critical condition. The large volume shifts associated with haemodialysis have also been implicated in the onset of NOMI and it has been

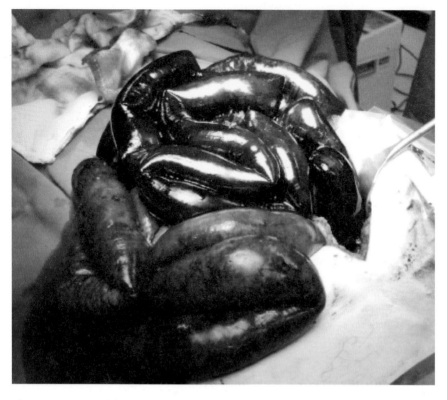

Fig. 4 An 82-year-old man presented with sudden abdominal pain. Nearly all the small bowel and part of large bowel were resected but the patient died in the postoperative period.

shown that 9–20% of deaths amongst patients on haemodialysis are attributable to NOMI.[4] Because bowel perfusion, similar to cerebral perfusion, is preserved in the setting of hypotension, NOMI represents a failure of autoregulation. Many vasoactive drugs may cause regional vasoconstriction, such as digitalis, cocaine, diuretics and vasopressin. Gross pathological arterial or venous occlusions are not observed in patients with NOMI. Ischaemia may not manifest itself for many hours, or even days.

Mesenteric venous thrombosis (MVT)

MVT is an infrequent condition occurring in only 5–10% of patients presenting with AMI. Frequently (*i.e.* > 80% of the time), it is the result of a process which increases a patient's propensity to coagulate within the mesenteric circulation (*i.e.* secondary MVT). Primary MVT occurs in the absence of any identifiable predisposing factor. In the past, a cause for MVT was found in < 50% of cases; now, multiple predisposing conditions have been identified with a cause now determined in 80–90% of cases (Table 1).[5] MVT may occur after ligation of the portal vein, or the superior mesenteric vein as part of 'damage-control surgery' for severe penetrating abdominal injuries. MVT often affects a much younger population. The chronic form of SMV thrombosis may manifest as oesophageal varices bleeding.

157

Table 1 Conditions associated with mesenteric venous thrombosis

Haematological/hypercoaguable states
        Sickle cell anaemia
        Polycythaemia vera
        Thrombosis
        Anti-thrombin III deficiency
        Protein C or protein S deficiency
        Factor V Leiden mutation (activated protein C resistance)
        Lupus anticoagulant
        Pregnancy
        Hepatic cirrhosis
        Congestive splenomegaly

Inflammatory conditions
        Peritonitis
        Cholangitis
        Pancreatitis
        Diverticulitis/appendicitis
        Intra-abdominal abscess
        Inflammatory bowel disease

Miscellaneous/general
        Ascaris lumbricoides infection
        Blunt abdominal trauma
        Decompression sickness
        Oestrogen-based medication

In summary, the mortality rate during the last 15 years from all causes of AMI has averaged 71%, with a range of 59–93%. Once bowel wall infarction has occurred, the mortality rate is as high as 90%. Survivors of mesenteric resection face significant, long-term morbidity due to a reduced intestinal mucosal surface available for absorption.

AMI can develop suddenly or slowly, with a progression over days. Classic symptoms of AMI include acute abdominal pain (out of proportion to the physical examination), with gut 'emptying' at the onset of pain. Bloody diarrhoea is a result of mucosal shedding and, usually, is a sign of advanced ischaemia.

Key point 2

- Overall, the mortality rate during the last 15 years from all causes of AMI has averaged 71%, with a range of 59–93%). Once whole bowel infarction has occurred, the mortality rate is as high as 90%.

CHRONIC MESENTERIC ISCHAEMIA

CMI is usually as a result of end-stage atherosclerosis (in the vast majority of cases). The prevalence of atherosclerosis increases with age, although somewhat unusually, there is a preponderance of CMI amongst females. The majority suffer also, from coronary artery and peripheral vascular disease elsewhere. Table 2 outlines the aetiology of CMI.

Table 2 Conditions underlying chronic mesenteric ischaemia

• Atherosclerosis (95% of cases)
• Neurofibromatosis
• Fibromuscular hyperplasia
• Aortic/visceral dissection
• Radiation therapy
• Connective tissue disease
• Cocaine abuse
• Antiphospholipid syndrome
• Behcet's disease
• Thromboangitis obliterans
• Takayasu's arteritis

CMI arises from severe stenosis, or occlusive disease affecting the origin of two or more of the three vessels mentioned above. However, if there is a poorly developed collateral circulation, even single-vessel disease can cause symptoms.

In about 50% of patients, the clinical presentation of CMI is identified by a triad comprising post-prandial abdominal pain ('abdominal angina'), 'food fear' and progressive weight loss. Other presenting signs or symptoms include gastritis, stomach ulceration, gastroparesis and diarrhoea. Emaciation may be evident in advanced cases and an abdominal bruit can be heard in up to 70% of patients.

Key point 3
- Chronic mesenteric ischaemia arises from severe stenosis, or occlusive disease affecting the origin of two or more of the three vessels.

ASSESSMENT

LABORATORY TESTS

Clinical laboratory findings are associated with patients with established AMI and often are not helpful in identifying patients sufficiently early to allow intervention which might significantly improve outcome. On admission, 75% of patients with AMI have a leukocytosis > 15,000 cells/mm^3 and approximately 50% have a metabolic acidosis. Additional late findings include a raised serum and peritoneal fluid amylase, raised serum D-lactate levels and a bacteraemia (arising from bacterial translocation across compromised bowel). Recently, a small study assessed the use of serum D-dimer levels in patients with AMI and found them to be elevated in all cases regardless of aetiology.[6] Generally, these biological parameters are not abnormal in CMI; hence, these tests are not helpful in identifying CMI.

Table 3 Ability of duplex ultrasonography to determine a 70% stenosis[14]

	Coeliac artery	Superior mesenteric artery
Sensitivity	87%	92%
Specificity	80%	96%
Positive predictive value	63%	80%
Negative predictive value	94%	99%
Overall accuracy	82%	96%

RADIOLOGICAL INVESTIGATIONS

Duplex ultrasonography

This is a non-invasive test which can be useful in evaluating patients with CMI. There are no universal criteria for grading coeliac and SMA stenoses, but a peak systolic velocity of over 200 cm/s for the coeliac artery, and over 275 cm/s for the SMA, in a fasting patient, suggests a 70% stenosis. In the hands of an experienced sonographer, duplex ultrasonography of the mesenteric vasculature is a valuable tool and should be considered to be the initial imaging modality of choice in a patient with presumed CMI (Fig. 5 and Table 3).[7]

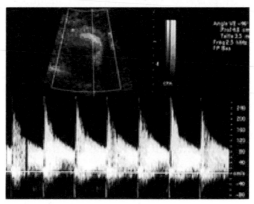

Fig. 5 A 45-year-old woman with abdominal pain immediately after a meal. Duplex scanning identified a significant stenosis of SMA and coeliac arteries.

Computed tomography (CT)

This is another non-invasive method of imaging the mesenteric vessels. Advances in this form of investigation (for example, multiple detector-row CT) has allowed radiologists to achieve satisfactory imaging of at least the proximal portion of the three main vessels. The ability to assess the degree of stenosis is inferior to that of the prevailing gold standard, catheter angiography. Therefore, CT is not the modality of choice for detecting those vascular abnormalities associated with CMI.

CT is useful in identifying the sequelae of AMI. Unfortunately, however, the early signs of AMI are relatively non-specific and the late signs accompany necrotic bowel.[8] A retrospective study of CT scan results in patients with

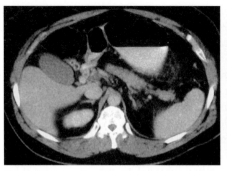
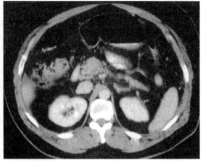

Fig. 6 CT scan of a 45-year-old patient who presented with abdominal pain. CT scan shows that SMV, portal and splenic veins are thrombosed. The patient was treated successfully with small bowel resection and kept on anticoagulant.

proven intestinal infarction showed specific findings in 39% of patients and non-specific findings in 35% of the cohort.[9] Other studies on the value of CT scanning in suspected AMI have demonstrated sensitivities ranging from 26–64%.[10] Early signs include bowel wall thickening and luminal dilatation. Late signs include pneumatosis coli (air in the bowel wall) and mesenteric/portal venous gas, both almost pathogenomonic of necrotic bowel. Contrast-enhanced CT scanning has established itself as the technique of choice for diagnosing acute MVT as it readily identifies the lack of opacification associated with an intraluminal thrombus (Fig. 6).

Catheter angiography and magnetic resonance angiography

Biplanar aortography remains the criterion standard test for the mesenteric vessels. Because the vessels emerge from the anterior wall of the aorta, the ostia are optimally visualised in a lateral projection. The presence of collaterals provides a clue to the underlying diagnosis of NOMI, despite the fact that stenoses or occlusions are best visualised with this form of high-quality imaging (Fig. 7). In the evaluation and correct diagnosis of splanchnic vessel

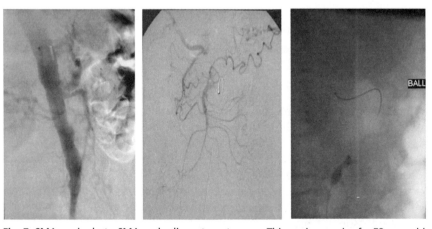

Fig. 7 SMA angioplasty, SMA and celiac artery stenoses. This angiogram is of a 52-year-old women who presented with abdominal pain 1–2 hours after a meal. Angiogram shows significant stenoses in both SMA and celiac arteries. She was treated successfully with angioplasty and stents.

disease, catheter angiography is superior to magnetic resonance angiography (MRA), with an overall accuracy of 94% versus 88%.[11] Furthermore, a recent review article suggests that MRA image resolution is too low for reliable assessment of the IMA.[12]

Selective mesenteric angiography and digital subtraction angiography (DSA) remain the investigations of choice for CMI and AMI. They can identify NOMI and provide important pre-operative information for mesenteric bypass surgery. Although routine angiography has decreased the mortality rate (without an increase in complications) in many series,[13] the role of pre-operative angiography is controversial in patients suspected of AMI and those with peritoneal signs. One surgical perspective is that performing angiography delays surgical treatment for critically ill patients and considering that positive angiographic findings are sometimes inconsistent, prompt surgical exploration has been advocated instead.

If emergency angiography has been performed, one or more filling defects with partial or complete flow obstruction may be seen. On this investigatory background, a decision on appropriate management must be made. Factors that should be taken into account are: (i) whether the embolus is in the SMA proximal to the ileocolic artery (major embolus), or more distally (minor embolus); (ii) whether the embolus is partially or completely occlusive; and (iii) whether or not there are signs of peritonitis.

Key point 4

- In emergency, CT angiography is the test of choice. There is no place for duplex scanning in the acute setting but this can be used in chronic conditions supported with conventional angiogram.

MANAGING ACUTE MESENTERIC ISCHAEMIA

Since most patients present with an acute abdomen, they will be subjected to routine assessment which includes basic blood tests and plain X-rays. If the diagnosis remains uncertain, then a CT scan should be performed. The CT scan will be able to identify ischaemic bowel and also to assess both the SMA and SMV.

SMV THROMBOSIS

SMV thrombosis alone, or combined with portal or renal vein thrombosis, could present with an acute abdomen. Presence of free air or septicaemia will necessitate laparotomy.

In the absence of peritonitis, no surgery is required, but full heparinisation and careful monitoring of all patients is essential. This should be maintained for a minimum of 7 days whilst concomitantly starting oral anticoagulation with warfarin or coumadin. During this time, the patient should be carefully monitored. More CT scanning may be required. Oral anti-coagulation should be continued for up to 6 months.

If the abdominal pain continues and anticoagulation is ineffective then laparotomy should be planned.

During exploration, the viability of bowel and extension of any ischaemic changes should be assessed. If bowel resection is required, any anastomosis should be deferred. It is essential to continue heparinisation for 7–10 days postoperatively as this has been shown to reduce the thrombotic recurrence rate from 25% to 13% and the mortality rate from 50% to 13%.[14]

Key point 5

- In SMV thrombosis, conservative treatment in the form of anti-coagulation and close monitoring is the first line of management. In case of deterioration, laparotomy should be performed.

MANAGEMENT OF AMAE AND AMAT

Once the diagnosis of SMA occlusion in the presence of an acute abdomen is established on CT scanning, then laparotomy should be performed. In surgery, when multifocal ischaemic changes of bowel is identified without an obvious perforation, or peritoneal soiling, exploration of the SMA should be performed. If the aetiology is embolic, a proximal pulse may be felt and an embolectomy should be attempted. Otherwise, in the case of thrombosis (where no pulse will be palpable and as thrombectomy is unlikely to be durable), a bypass should be performed. If the embolectomy is unsuccessful, then the surgeon should proceed to bypass surgery. Two options are available – either antegrade or retrograde bypass using either vein, or a synthetic graft. Preferentially, a reversed vein graft is used, especially if bowel resection is required, to minimise graft infection. A 'second look' laparotomy should be planned.

When most of the small bowel and the large bowel to the mid part of the transverse colon are gangrenous, a major bowel resection is required; thus, no revascularisation bypass is needed. These patients are likely to require life-long parenteral nutrition.

Occasionally, the patient presents with an acute event on top of atherosclerotic disease of SMA which is associated with a limited length of a gangrenous bowel segment found with major peritoneal soiling. In these cases, it is reasonable to resect the bowel, with stoma formation; a 'second-look' operation should be planned for the following 24 hours. During this period, all patients should be kept on heparin infusion and an angiogram should be performed to identify any proximal SMA stenosis, which can be pre-treated by balloon angioplasty. In this fails, bypass surgery should be performed during the second-look operation.

In the absence of peritoneal signs, infusions of vasodilators or thrombolytic agents have been used with some success. Although not a standard treatment, intra-arterial Papaverine has been used to achieve vasodilation, at a continuous rate of 30–60 mg/h. This has been done in selected instances (for example, minor emboli, poor surgical candidates, or in the absence of peritoneal signs) by some groups for up to 5 days without complication. Similarly, thrombolytic agents have been used with varying success in this scenario with comparable restrictions (partial occlusion, < 12 h history).[15,16]

NON-OCCLUSIVE MESENTERIC ISCHAEMIA (NOMI)

Frequently, in the case of NOMI, the high mortality rates are attributed to a delay in diagnosis because of non-specific symptoms compared with other types of AMI. The symptomatology of NOMI has been explored by Reinus *et al.*[17] who identified that it is often preceded by a gradual onset of crampy, peri-umbilical pain progressing to constant pain. The patients at highest risk have predisposing factors such as diabetes mellitus, hypertension and hyperlipidaemia (all associated with atherosclerosis). A high index of suspicion is a prerequisite to allow appropriate investigation, as angiography is the only technique available to diagnose NOMI prior to the occurrence of bowel infarction. Currently, four criteria are used in this diagnosis:[18] (i) narrowing of the origins of the SMA branches; (ii) radiological irregularities in these branches; (iii) spasm of the mesenteric arcades; and (iv) impaired filling of the intramural vessels.

Using these principles, NOMI has been identified before infarction (with a lack of peritoneal signs); hence, it is possible to use intra-arterial Papaverine to relieve vasoconstriction, prevent progressive ischaemia and avoid laparotomy. In series where Papaverine has been used in this way following angiography, significant reductions in mortality have been achieved.[19] Papaverine alone may achieve the

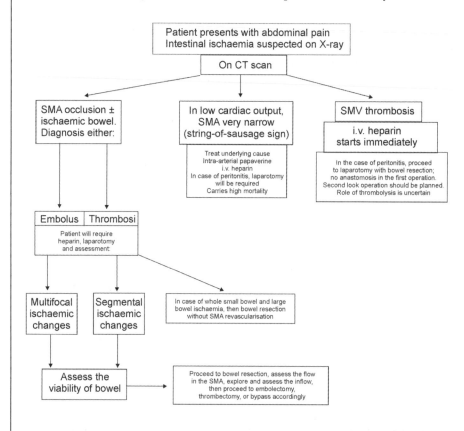

Fig. 8 Management of acute mesenteric ischaemia. In these cases; i.v. heparin is needed and a second-look laparotomy is required except in the case of a major bowel resection.

desired result. However, the presence of peritoneal signs, or a prolonged ischaemic time (> 12 h) may indicate the requirement for laparotomy and bowel resection. Papaverine should be administered continuously before, during and after surgery.[8] Preservation of 'questionable' bowel is recommended as re-exploration has demonstrated that Papaverine can have a dramatic effect on bowel of dubious viability. Boley *et al.*[20] have reported that this treatment algorithm may limit the length of bowel resected to one metre in up to 75% of patients with AMI (Fig. 8).

Key point 6

- In acute splenic mesenteric artery ischaemia, embolectomy should be performed; based on its outcome, the surgeon should proceed to by-pass surgery.

MANAGING CHRONIC MESENTERIC ISCHAEMIA

SURGICAL MANAGEMENT

Patients with proven symptomatic CMI benefit from surgical intervention, but this is associated with a greater risk of complications than with other forms of elective surgery. Surgical treatment involves revascularisation of the stenotic or occluded mesenteric vessels using autogenous, or prosthetic grafts. The superiority enjoyed by donor vein elsewhere in vascular surgery does not extend to mesenteric reconstruction.[21]

Inflow may be provided to the coeliac axis or SMA either from the supra-coeliac aorta (antegrade reconstruction) or the infra-renal aorta/common iliac artery (retrograde reconstruction). Advocates of antegrade reconstruction suggest that because the bypass is positioned in the direction of normal blood flow, anastomotic turbulence is avoided, thereby reducing the likelihood of progressive atherosclerotic disease or thrombosis. It has been proposed that this form of reconstruction is also less prone to kinking and consequent thrombosis. Despite this, proponents of the retrograde bypass maintain that they provide a comparable long-term prevention of recurrence.[22] When the disease affects all three vessels, it has been shown that complete revascularisation results in a much lower recurrence rate (11%) than when only one stenotic vessel is bypassed (50%).[23]

Table 4 Results of recent studies examining revascularisation for chronic mesenteric ischaemia

	Patients	Mortality	Follow-up (yrs)	Late patency
Johnston *et al.* (1995)[26]	21	0	NA	86%
Taylor *et al.* (2000)[27]	84	11%	11	95%
Foley *et al.* (2000)[28]	49	12%	9	79%
Park *et al.* (2002)[3]	98	5.1%	5	92%

Postoperatively, some patients experience psychological difficulty in resuming a normal diet and, frequently, total parenteral nutrition is employed in this phase of a patient's treatment.

ENDOVASCULAR MANAGEMENT OF CMI

There is very little information available pertaining to the endovascular treatment of CMI. There have been two studies directly comparing endovascular repair and open surgery. However, as neither provide (level I) evidence, we cannot draw any definitive conclusions as to which method of revascularisation is superior. Nonetheless , both studies indicate that surgery is the more durable option despite having a greater incidence of major systemic complications. In a study by Kasirajan et al.,[24] long-term patency (3 years) was superior in the surgery group (87% versus 66%). Rose et al.[25] found that the recurrence rate in the endovascular group was 33% as opposed to 12% in the open surgery group.

Despite the apparently better patency results with surgery, it must be remembered that patients with CMI have significant co-morbidity and the choice of procedure must always be tailored to specific circumstances.

Key point 7

- Despite the apparently better patency results with surgery, it must be remembered that patients with chronic mesenteric ischaemia have significant co-morbidity and the choice of procedure must always be tailored to specific circumstances.

CONCLUSIONS

Ischaemic injury to the gastrointestinal tract is a potentially catastrophic event and mortality rates remain high. The presenting signs and symptoms are frequently non-specific and accurate diagnosis requires a high index of suspicion. This may be aided by acknowledging that the specific sub-population affected by AMI is one at high-risk, with a significant history of systemic vascular disease. Therefore, an aggressive diagnostic schematic should be employed. Certain patients, such as those on haemodialysis, have an even stronger predisposition to ischaemic events and intestinal ischaemia should always be suspected in such patients reporting even vague abdominal symptoms. If the diagnosis is considered sufficiently early, mesenteric angiography should be attempted with a view to pharmaco-angiographic treatment (in selected cases). When obvious peritoneal signs necessitate surgery, a practical, but prudent, approach is mandated which should be accompanied by appropriate use of 'second-look' laparotomy.

CMI is a rare progressive disease entity requiring vascular expertise in its evaluation and management. Currently, open surgery offers the best results. However, the prevalence of significant co-morbid disease in CMI patients suggests that endovascular repair should perhaps be preferentially offered to those with a high surgical risk profile.

Key points for clinical practice

- Acute mesenteric ischaemia has an in-hospital mortality rate of 59–93% while chronic mesenteric ischaemia has an excellent prognosis, with low operative mortality and long-term survival rates of 50–60%.

- Overall, the mortality rate during the last 15 years from all causes of acute mesenteric ischaemia has averaged 71%, with a range of 59–93%. Once bowel wall infarction has occurred, the mortality rate is as high as 90%.

- Chronic mesenteric ischaemia arises from severe stenosis, or occlusive disease affecting the origin of two or more of the three vessels.

- In emergency, CT angiography is the test of choice. There is no place for duplex scanning in the acute setting but this can be used in chronic conditions supported with conventional angiogram.

- In SMV thrombosis, conservative treatment in the form of anticoagulation and close monitoring is the first line of management. In case of deterioration, laparotomy should be performed.

- In acute splenic mesenteric artery ischaemia, embolectomy should be performed; based on its outcome, the surgeon should proceed to by-pass surgery.

- Despite the apparently better patency results with surgery, it must be remembered that patients with chronic mesenteric ischaemia have significant co-morbidity and the choice of procedure must always be tailored to specific circumstances.

References

1. Cokkinis AJ. *Mesenteric Vascular Occlusion*. London: Baillière, Tindall and Cox, 1926.
2. Brandt LJ, Boley SJ and American Gastrointestinal Association. AGA technical review on intestinal ischaemia. *Gastroenterolgy* 2000; **118**: 954–968.
3. Park WM, Cherry Jr KJ, Chua HK *et al*. Current results of open revascularisation for chronic mesenteric ischaemia: a standard for comparison. *J Vasc Surg* 2002; **35**: 853–859.
4. Yashuhara H. Acute mesenteric ischaemia: the challenge of gastroenterology. *Surg Today* 2005; **35**: 185–195.
5. Rhee RY, Globviczki P, Mendonca CT *et al*. Mesenteric venous thrombosis: still a lethal disease in the 1990s. *J Vasc Surg* 1994; **20**: 688–697.
6. Acosta S, Nilsson TK, Bjork M. Preliminary study of D-dimer as a possible marker of acute bowel ischaemia. *Br J Surg* 2001; **88**: 385–388.
7. Moneta GL, Lee RW, Yeager RA. Mesenteric duplex scanning: a blinded prospective study. *J Vasc Surg* 1993; **17**: 79–84.
8. Bartnicke B, Balfe D. CT appearance of intestinal ischemia and intramural hemorrhage. *Radiol Clin North Am* 1994; **32**: 845–860.
9. Smerud M, Johnson C, Stephens D. Diagnosis of bowel infarction: a comparison of plain films and CT scans in 23 cases. *AJR Am J Roentgenol* 1990; **154**: 99–103.

10. Alpern MB, Glazer GM, Francis IR. Ischemic or infarcted bowel: CT findings. *Radiology* 1988; **166**: 149–152.

11. Ernst O, Asnar V, Sergent G *et al*. Comparing contrast-enhanced breath-hold MR angiography and conventional angiography in the evaluation of mesenteric circulation. *AJR Am J Roentgenol* 2000; **174**: 433–439.

12. Vosshenrich R, Fischer U. Contrast-enhanced MR angiography of abdominal vessels: is there still a role for angiography? *Eur Radiol* 2002; **12**: 218–230.

13. Schneider TA, Longo WE, Ure T, Vernava III AM. Mesenteric ischaemia: acute arterial syndromes. *Dis Colon Rectum* 1994; **37**: 1163–1174.

14. Grieshop RJ, Dalsing MC, Cikrit DF *et al*. Acute mesenteric venous thrombosis: revisited in a time of diagnostic clarity. *Am Surg* 1991; **57**: 573–577 (discussion 578).

15. Gallego AM, Ramirez P, Rodriguez JM *et al*. Role of urokinase in the superior mesenteric artery embolism. *Surgery* 1996; **120**: 111–113.

16. Simo G, Echenaguisia AJ, Camunez F, Turegano F, Cabrera A, Urbano J. Superior mesenteric artery embolism: local fibrinolytic treatment with urokinase. *Radiology* 1997; **204(3)**: 775–779.

17. Reinus JF, Brandt LJ, Boley SJ. Ischemic disease of the bowel. *Gastroenterol Clin North Am* 1990; **19**: 319–340.

18. Bakal CW, Sprayregen S, Wolf EL. Radiology in intestinal ischemia. Angiographic diagnosis and management. *Surg Clin North Am* 1992; **72**: 125–141.

19. Boley SJ, Sprayregen S, Siegelmann SS, Veith FJ. Initial results from an aggressive approach to acute mesenteric ischaemia. *Surgery* 1977; **82**: 848–855.

20. Boley SJ, Sprayregen S, Veith FJ *et al*. An aggressive roentgenologic and surgical approach to acute mesenteric ischemia. In: Nyhus LM. (ed) *Surgery Annual*. New York: Appleton-Century-Crofts, 1973; 355.

21. Moawad J, McKinsey JF, Wyble CW, Bassiouny HS, Schwartz LB, Gewertz BL. Current results of surgical therapy for chronic mesenteric ischaemia. *Arch Surg* 1997; **132**: 613–619.

22. Gentile AT, Moneta GL, Taylor Jr LM, Park TC, McConnell DB, Porter JM. Isolated bypass to the superior mesenteric artery for intestinal ischemia. *Arch Surg* 1994; **129**: 926–931.

23. Hollier LH, Bernatz PE, Pairolero PC, Payne WS, Osmundson PJ. Surgical management of chronic intestinal ischemia: a reappraisal. *Surgery* 1981; **90**: 940–946.

24. Kasirajan K, O'Hara PJ, Gray BH *et al*. Chronic mesenteric ischemia: open surgery versus percutaneous angioplasty and stenting. *J Vasc Surg* 2001; **33**: 63–71.

25. Rose SC, Quiglet TM, Raker EJ. Revascularization for chronic mesenteric ischaemia: comparison of operative arterial bypass grafting and percutaneous transluminal angioplasty. *J Vasc Intervent Radiol* 1995; **6**: 339–349.

26. Johnston K, Lindsay T, Walker P. Mesenteric arterial bypass grafts: early and late results and suggested surgical approach for chronic and acute mesenteric ischemia. *Surgery* 1995; **118**: 1–7.

27. Taylor L, Moneta G, Porter J. Treatment of chronic visceral ischema. In: Rutherford RB (ed) Vascular Surgery Philadelphia: WB Saunders, 2000: 1532–1541.

28. Foley M, Moneta G, Abou-Zamzam A. Revascularization of the superior mesenteric artery alone for treatment of intestinal ischemia. *J Vasc Surg* 2000; **32**: 37–47.

Rovan E. D'Souza Daryll M. Baker

13

Complications of arteriovenous haemodialysis fistulas

Complications of haemodialysis access have been the Achilles' tendon for patients on haemodialysis and for the treating health personnel. Of patients with vascular access, 15–25% require hospitalisation for vascular access complications.[1] Hospitalisation rates for fistula complications are higher in patients with diabetes mellitus and of black race.[2–4] Lesser complications and better patency with arteriovenous fistula (AVF) compared to arteriovenous graft (AVG) fistula or tunnelled catheter access has made AVF the preferred vascular access.[5] An ever expanding haemodialysis service has made vascular access for haemodialysis a common procedure but with associated complications which are discussed in this chapter. The common complications of an arteriovenous fistula are summarised in Table 1.

BLEEDING

IMMEDIATE OR EARLY

Early haemorrhage could be due to bleeding tendency in uraemic patients,[6] severed vessels during dissection or an anastomotic bleed. Patients having vascular access procedures should have bleeding and clotting assessed pre-operatively. Meticulous haemostasis is of paramount importance. Anastomotic bleed is not a common problem unless there is a technical flaw.

Rovan E. D'Souza FRCS(Glasg.) MS DNB
Senior Clinical Fellow, Department of Vascular Surgery, Royal Free Hospital, Pond Street, London
NW3 2QH, UK
E-mail: rovand@hotmail.com

Daryll M. Baker PhD FRCS (for correspondence)
Consultant Surgeon, Department of Vascular Surgery, Royal Free Hampstead NHS Trust, Pond St,
London NW3 2QG, UK
E-mail: baker@freevas.demon.co.uk

Table 1 Common complications of an arteriovenous fistula

- Bleeding
- Thrombosis
- Acute ischaemia and steal syndrome
- Ischaemic monomelic neuropathy
- Carpal tunnel syndrome
- Venous hypertension
- Aneurysmal dilatation of the vein
- Pseudoaneurysm
- High output cardiac failure
- Sterile fluid collections (haematoma, seroma)
- Infection
- Pulmonary hypertension

DELAYED OR LATE

Delayed or late occurrence of bleeding complications in a vascular access is often encountered with a puncture site. Use of inappropriately large calibre cannula (more than 18-G) for dialysis is a common cause. Coagulopathy and use of heparin during dialysis predispose these patients to haemorrhagic episodes. Adequate pressure applied over the puncture site after removal of the cannula would prevent this complication. Excessive puncture site bleeding is associated with stenosis in the outflow vein secondary to high venous pressure distal to the stenosis. Duplex scan and angiography or MR venography will delineate the lesion. Angioplasty of the stenotic segment would prevent further recurrence and will prevent thrombosis of vascular access and venous hypertension. Rarely, accidental injury to the vascular access may cause bleeding from the site.

Key point 1

- Native arteriovenous fistula placed as distal as possible yields best results with respect to longevity and complications.

THROMBOSIS

EARLY THROMBOSIS (< 30 DAYS)

Early thrombosis may be due to faulty technique of anastomosis, twisted or acutely angulated outflow vein, low cardiac output, diseased inflow artery and stenosis or occlusion in the outflow vein and, rarely, a hypercoagulable state. Early vascular access thrombosis is reported to be higher with radiocephalic fistula at the wrist especially in diabetic patients compared to elbow fistulas and arteriovenous grafts.[7,8] The role of aspirin, clopidogrel and heparin in improving patency rates of fistulas is not well established. Dipyridamole and fish oil[7] have been reported to improve patency of vascular access in small randomised studies. Dipyridamole is a potent inhibitor of fibromuscular dysplasia.[9]

Persistent or recurrent thrombosis may prompt investigation for a hypercoagulable state. Most patients with chronic renal failure have associated ischaemic heart disease with low cardiac output further compounded by hypovolaemia. This may result in a low flow across the fistula causing thrombosis. Diseased peripheral arteries are another common association in these patients. Thus, patients considered for AVF or AVG construction should be examined and investigated accordingly and optimised pre-operatively. A routine pre-operative history and clinical examination, which would include the Allen's test, is recommended. Allen's test, in view of its wide inter-observer differences,[10] should be used with caution. A pressure difference of more than 20 mmHg on either upper limbs should raise suspicion of decreased blood flow in the arm with the lower pressure. Duplex scan of the target artery and vein has been shown to improve success rates of the fistula. Radial artery and cephalic vein diameter at the wrist of at least 1.6–2.0 mm[7,12,13] and subclavian venous flow of at least 400 ml/min[14] pre-operatively have been shown to yield better vascular access patency. Diabetic patients and those with peripheral vascular disease are at a higher risk of access thrombosis.[15]

DELAYED OR LATE THROMBOSIS (> 30 DAYS)

Delayed thrombosis of AVF/AVG may be due to stenosis in either the inflow artery or the outflow vein, low blood pressure secondary to cardiac or non-cardiac causes, faulty technique at cannulation or during removal of the dialysis cannula. Stenosis in the outflow vein is the commonest cause of thrombosis and typically occurs within the first 4 cm from the anastomosis with the artery, probably due to intimal trauma caused by a high pressure and turbulent flow and subsequent smooth muscle hyperplasia and fibrosis. Intimal hyperplasia is seen at the graft–vein interface.[9] Mutagens such as platelet derived growth factors (PDGFs), thromboxane or other mediators[9] released at the venepuncture sites may play a role in the pathogenesis. Exogenously administered erythropoietin has also been implicated.[16] Vascular access must be monitored for development of inflow or outflow stenosis. A routine surveillance programme, early diagnosis and timely intervention improve vascular access patency[9,10] and reduce morbidity. Cannulation by experienced staff and adherence to recommended techniques are extremely important.

The methods used to monitor vascular access are: (i) physical examination; (ii) recirculation; (iii) venous pressure measurements; and (iv) graft blood flow.

Physical examination
Prolonged bleeding from puncture site, absence of pulse or thrill beyond a certain point, abnormally dilated or aneurysmal outflow vein are all indicators of a stenosis in the outflow vein.

Recirculation
A recirculation value of 10% or more should be investigated for developing stenosis.[1] Recirculation in vascular access is a condition where the blood from the arterial cannula flows through the dialyser instead of flowing into the outflow vein and towards the heart, the dialysed blood returns into the arterial

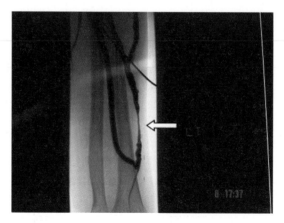

cannula through the vascular access and back into the dialyser. Recirculation is measured using urea or the newer indicator dilution methods.

Venous pressure measurements

Dynamic and static pressures within a graft or vein measured with the patient connected to the haemodialysis machine are an indirect assessment of vascular access flow. Static pressure is more sensitive in predicting a stenosis.[7] However, venous pressure is a relatively late predictor of impending thrombosis.[1,9]

Graft blood flow

Blood flow measurement using Doppler ultrasound or the ultrasound dilution technique is reported to be accurate in early detection of stenosis[17,18] but is observer-dependent. A wide range of criteria using Doppler ultrasound have been described with a vascular access flow ranging from 200–750 ml/min.[10] El Minshawy et al.[18] found a vascular access flow of less than 200 ml/min, resistivity index (PSV–DSV/PSV) of less than 0.1 and a peak velocity of more than 1.5 m/s to be predictive of stenosis . Kim et al.[19] have reported AVF thrombosis at a flow less than 350 ml/min. In case of AVGs, a flow rate of 600 ml/min or less may predict stenosis.[9] According to the NKF-DOQI guidelines,[1] patients with a vascular access flow of 1000 ml/min that has decreased by more than 25% over 4 months or a flow less than 600 ml/min should be referred for a fistulogram (Fig. 1).

Fig. 1 Fistulogram of end-to-side radiocephalic fistula showing stenosis in the outflow vein.

TREATMENT OF THROMBOSED VASCULAR ACCESS

Traditionally, a thrombosed graft would be treated by surgical thrombectomy. Advances in interventional radiology in the past decade have seen an increasing number of patients being treated with percutaneous techniques. The advantage is that the entire anatomy of the inflow artery and the outflow vein, as well as the graft when present, are studied and simultaneously treated. The options available to the radiologist in the treatment of thrombosed or dysfunctional vascular access are summarised in Table 2.

There is no evidence to support or denounce any one technique. The key to prolonged patency is early identification and successful treatment of all lesions

Table 2 Options available to the radiologist in the treatment of thrombosed or dysfunctional vascular access

- Angioplasty + tPA or reptilase infusion
- Stenting of a stenosis
- Thrombolysis (tPA or urokinase)
- Pulse spray pharmacomechanical thrombolysis
- Balloon thrombectomy techniques
- Mechanical thrombectomy

on the arterial and venous side and the complete removal of arterial thrombus, if any. Brachytherapy or endovascular radiotherapy, successfully used in the prevention of restenosis following coronary angioplasty, is being tried to reduce the intimal and fibromuscular hyperplasia at the vein–graft interface and in the treatment of stenosis in the outflow vein after angioplasty.[20,21]

Key point 2

- Thrombosis of the vascular access is the commonest complication and the role of anti-platelets is not yet established.

STEAL SYNDROME AND DISTAL ISCHAEMIA

Steal syndrome and ischaemia of the hand (Fig. 2) is caused by preferential blood flow into the vascular access. A 40% reduction in blood flow to the thumb has been reported after a radiocephalic fistula at the wrist, but most patients are asymptomatic.[22] The incidence of symptomatic steal is reported to be 1.7% with wrist fistulas and up to 8% with elbow fistulas.[23] Allen's test, supplemented by Doppler arterial study and digital brachial pressure index of less than 0.6 will identify patients at risk of developing steal.[24] Patients with steal may have either a low-flow or a high-flow fistula. Low flow occurs when a diseased inflow radial artery causes diversion of blood flow from the ulnar artery into the fistula. In a high-flow fistula blood from the radial and ulnar artery flows preferentially into the fistula causing ischaemia of the digits. Proximal AVFs are more prone to the steal phenomenon as the outflow vein is larger with higher distensibilty. Presence of distal ulnar and radial artery disease would worsen the situation.

Clinical presentation includes pain distal to the fistula, diminished or altered sensation (paraesthesia or numbness), pale and cold hand, absent or diminished pulses, poor capillary refill, diminished movements or digital ulcers and gangrene. The differential diagnosis of steal syndrome is acute thrombosis of the artery causing critical ischaemia. Compression of the fistula will relieve symptoms if due to steal.

Confirmation of diagnosis

Doppler scan – Measurement of the flow by saline dilution technique is useful in differentiating a high-flow from a low-flow fistula and in ruling out acute thrombosis of the access vis-à-vis the inflow artery.

Angiography – Angiography before and after occlusion of the access will establish the aetiology and assist in further intervention.

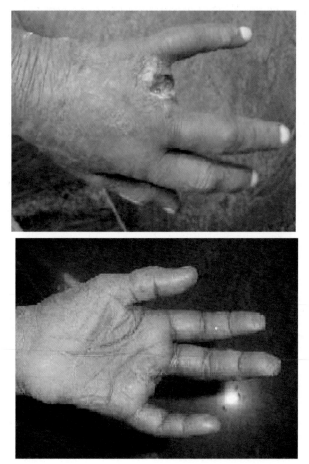

Fig. 2 Steal syndrome following a brachio-basilic fistula with loss of 4th digit and ischaemic finger tips.

Treatment

Angioplasty of the stenosed inflow radial artery may relieve symptoms thus preserving the fistula. Distal revascularisation and interval ligation (DRIL)[25] involves ligation of the inflow artery distal to the arteriovenous or artery-to-graft anastomosis and a vein bypass with the proximal anastomosis of the bypass being about 5 cm proximal to the fistula and the distal anastomosis being just distal to the ligation. This would preserve the fistula and restore vascularity to the ischaemic digits. In high flow AVFs, banding of the venous segment decreases flow in the fistula. The efficacy of this procedure is assessed by partially occluding the fistula to such an extent that the flow through the fistula is just optimum, as assessed with a sterile stethoscope for presence of a bruit or by duplex scan. This procedure initially preserves the access and improves distal perfusion but limits access patency.[26] The access is sacrificed if the above options fail and the limb is threatened.

ISCHAEMIC MONOMELIC NEUROPATHY(IMN)

This is a rare, but devastating, complication of arteriovenous access procedures. The pathogenesis of the condition is not clearly known but is thought to be due to ischaemia of the nerves secondary to reduced or altered flow through the vasa nervosum. It is characterised by acute, and usually irreversible, neurological dysfunction of the radial, ulnar and median nerves. The soft tissues of the hand as such are not ischaemic, differentiating this from vascular steal. Nerve conduction studies are useful in the diagnosis of unilateral cases. In bilateral diabetic neuropathy with super-added IMN, it is impossible to diagnose the latter. When the median nerve only is involved, it is difficult to differentiate it from carpel tunnel syndrome.

Diabetic, female patients with uraemia and patients with proximal fistulas seem to be at a higher risk. Symptoms occur within 24 h of the arteriovenous access procedure. The treatment options include flow-limiting banding or ligation, observation and aggressive physiotherapy. The treatment response is widely variable.

Carpal tunnel syndrome (CTS) is another neurological complication that occurs with vascular access. The pathogenesis is not known but thought to be secondary to venous compression of the median nerve, oedema, thickened carpal tissues, vascular steal and amyloid deposition and may not be a direct result of the vascular access. When CTS is suspected, the treatment should proceed towards decompression.

Immediate postoperative haematoma around the elbow may press on the median nerve and present with acute median nerve palsy. Evacuation of the haematoma and haemostasis give good results but may result in sacrificing the fistula.[27]

VENOUS HYPERTENSION

Venous hypertension in most patients with vascular access is asymptomatic. It can be painful and limb threatening. Patients with stenosis in the outflow vein anywhere from the arteriovenous anastomosis to the right atrium or paucity of venous collaterals and those with a side-to-side fistula develop this complication. The presentation may be mild-to-gross oedema that may lead to elephantiasis, bluish discoloration or hyperpigmentation of skin, finger tip ulcers, neuralgia or venous gangrene (Fig. 3A). Duplex scan and angiography are helpful in the assessment.

The treatment is angioplasty of the stenotic lesion, embolisation of the AVF or surgical ligation of the fistula. Many of these patients have had subclavian vein cannulation for temporary dialysis access or pacemaker insertion resulting in proximal venous stenosis (Fig. 3B & Fig. 4). Angioplasty is the best option for these patients.

HIGH-OUTPUT CARDIAC FAILURE

Cardiac failure following vascular access creation is rare;[28] fistulas around the elbow are more likely to cause this. Most patients with renal failure have impaired cardiac function secondary to pre-existing ischaemic heart disease or cardiomyopathy, fluid overload and anaemia. Patients with fistula flow rates

A

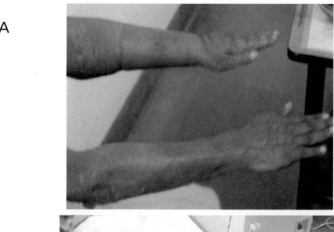

B

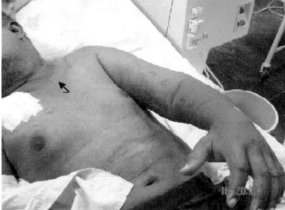

Fig. 3 (A) Oedema of the left forearm due to venous hypertension following a proximal radiocephalic fistula. (B) Oedema of the arm in a patient with radiocephalic fistula and left subclavian vein stenosis. Note the dilated veins in the neck.

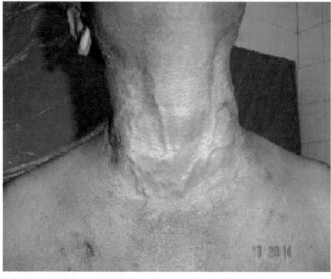

Fig. 4 Dilated veins in the neck and chest in a patient with brachiocephalic AVF suggestive of SVC occlusion.

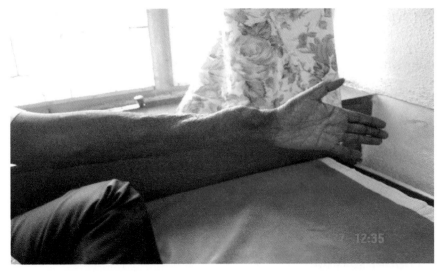

Fig. 5 Aneurysmal dilatation of outflow vein in a radiocephalic fistula.

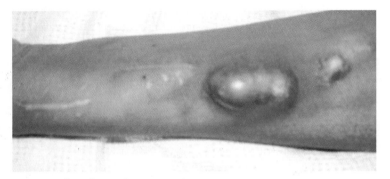

Fig. 6 Aneurysm of outflow vein at same site puncture.

of more than 1.5 l/min[29] and an access flow to cardiac output ratio higher than 0.3[30] are at high risk of high-output cardiac failure. Once diagnosed, a step graft or flow-limiting banding are methods to decrease flow across the fistula thereby decreasing the venous return to the heart. In severe cases, ligation of the fistula may be required.

ANEURYSMAL DILATATION OF THE VEIN OR GRAFT

Aneurysms of the outflow vein are a result of vessel wall destruction and replacement by biophysically inferior collagen (Figs 5 and 6). Repeated puncture of the same segment with scar formation also predisposes to the development of an aneurysm. Stenosis proximal to the aneurysm may be demonstrated by elevating the limb and looking for collapse of the segment proximal to the stenosis and persistence of the dilatation distal to it. Duplex scan and angiography will confirm the diagnosis and define the lesion. Untreated, these aneurysms may rupture, cause orthograde or retrograde embolism or get infected. Their course is usually benign and intervention is rarely indicated.[1] Aneurysms more than 2 cm in diameter or twice the lumen of the outflow vein need to be treated.

Treatment involves angioplasty of stenotic lesions and/or excision of aneurysms and end-to-end anastomosis. Long segment lesions may require excision of the vein and interposition vein or synthetic graft.

Key point 3 & 4

- Pre-operative assessment and surveillance program to screen for vascular access complications decrease morbidity and improves longevity of the vascular access.

- Endovascular procedures have made management of complications minimally invasive and quick.

PSEUDOANEURYSM

This complication occurs when inadequate pressure is applied to the puncture site in a graft fistula. Excessive pressure in the venous segment seconary to proximal stenosis requiring excessive compression at puncture sites is sometimes the cause (Fig. 7).

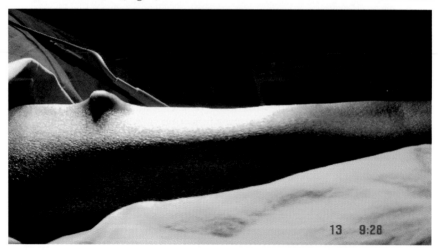

Fig. 7 Pseudoaneurysm at infected PTFE graft–vein anastomosis.

Indications for surgical intervention include rapid expansion, an aneurysm twice the diameter of the graft, possible or impending rupture, compromised overlying skin and infection. The treatment includes ultrasound-guided compression treatment, thrombin injection at the neck of the pseudoaneurysm, stent repair or surgical repair.[31,32] It may also be approached radiologically and embolised with coils.

STERILE FLUID COLLECTIONS AND HAEMATOMAS

Sterile fluid collections occur with graft fistulas due to fluid oozing from the graft surface. Seromas may occur when the vascular access procedure involves extensive dissection. Haematomas occur when adequate pressure is not applied over the puncture site and as a result of postoperative bleed as discussed earlier.

> ## Key point 5
>
> • Brachytherapy in the treatment of stenotic lesions looks promising.

INFECTION

Infection of vascular access is a major cause of morbidity and mortality. Access site infection is reported to be the cause in 48–73% of all bacteraemia in haemodialysis patients.[33] The incidence of vascular access infection is higher with tunnelled catheters and AVGs compared to native fistulas.

Occluded grafts have been reported to cause recurrent infection in haemodialysis patients. Immediate postoperative infection can be decreased by pre-operative prophylactic use of vancomycin.[34] The commonest organism implicated is *Staphylococcus* spp., which in addition to access site infection can cause metastatic infections. When an infective complication is suspected, empirical antimicrobial treatment is commenced determined by local guidelines and severity of illness. Long-term antibiotic treatment is required in these patients to prevent recurrence.

An abscess requires drainage after confirmation that there is no communication with the fistula (Figs 8 and 9). An infected graft should be removed to prevent progression of the infection. Strict adherence to guidelines in the care of vascular access and preference for a native fistula to a graft or tunnelled vascular access reduces this complication. Distant infections such as infective endocarditis have been reported in patients with infected grafts that are not excised.[35]

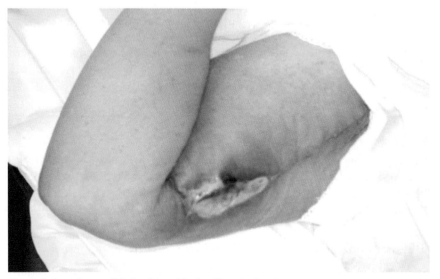

Fig. 8 Infected superficialised brachio-bacilic vein fistula.

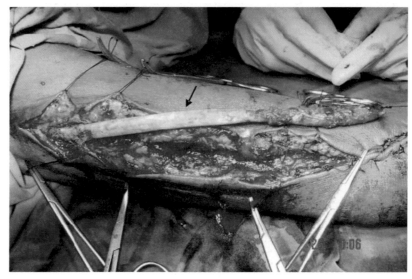

Fig. 9 Infected PTFE graft fistula in the forearm. Note the bare graft proximally which is typical of an infected graft.

Key point 6 & 7

- DRIL is a useful procedure when appropriately used in patients with steal.

- Cardiac complications such as high-output failure and pulmonary hypertension are rare but may occur with vascular access for haemodialysis.

PULMONARY HYPERTENSION

Pulmonary hypertension is reported in patients on haemodialysis. Nitric oxide (NO), endothelin-1 (ET-1) and the increased pulmonary blood flow caused by increased venous return leading to higher pulmonary vascular resistance are thought to play a role.[36] The vascular access may be just another factor and closure of the fistula is rarely required.

Key points for clinical practice

- Native arteriovenous fistula placed as distal as possible yields best results with respect to longevity and complications.

- Thrombosis of the vascular access is the commonest complication and the role of anti-platelets is not yet established.

- Pre-operative assessment and surveillance program to screen for vascular access complications decrease morbidity and improves longevity of the vascular access.   *(continued)*

Key points for clinical practice *(continued)*

- Endovascular procedures have made management of complications minimally invasive and quick.

- Brachytherapy in the treatment of stenotic lesions looks promising.

- DRIL is a useful procedure when appropriately used in patients with steal.

- Cardiac complications such as high-output failure and pulmonary hypertension are rare but may occur with vascular access for haemodialysis.

References

1. National Kidney Foundation. K/DOQI clinical practice guidelines for vascular access morbidity. *Am J Kidney Dis* 2001; **37 (Suppl 1)**: S137–S181.
2. Windus DW. Permanent vascular access: a nephrologist's view. *Am J Kidney Dis* 1993; **21**: 457–471.
3. Golledge J, Smith CJ, Emery J, Farrington K, Thompson HH. Outcome of primary radiocephalic fistulas for hemodialysis. *Br J Surg* 1999; **86**: 211–216.
4. Leapman SB, Boyle M, Pescovitz MD, Milgrom ML, Jindal RM, Filo RS. The arteriovenous fistula for hemodialysis access: gold standard or archaic relic? *Am Surg* 1996; **62**: 652–656.
5. Winsett OE, Wolma FJ. Complications of vascular access for hemodialysis. *South Med J* 1985; **78**: 513–517.
6. Salman S. Uremic bleeding: pathophysiology, diagnosis, and management. *Hosp Physician* 2001; 45–56,76.
7. Vassalotti JA, Falk A, Teodorescu V, Uribarri J. The multidisciplinary approach to hemodialysis vascular access at The Mount Sinai Hospital. *Mount Sinai J Med* 2004; **71**: 94–102.
8. Hakim R, Himmelfarb J. Hemodialysis access failure: a call to action. *Kidney Int* 1998: **54**: 1029–1040.
9. Schwab SJ, Butterly DW. Dialysis therapy. In: Massy SG, Glassock RJ. (eds) *Textbook of Nephrology*, 4th edn. Baltimore, MD: Lippincot William and Wilkins, 2001; 1480–1488.
10. Tessitore N, Bedogna V, Poli A. The role of surveillance in mature arteriovenous fistula management. *J Vasc Access* 2004; **5**: 57–61.
11. Cable DG, Mullany CJ, Schaff HV. The Allen test. *Ann Thor Surg* 1999; **67**: 876–877.
12. Wong V, Ward R, Taylor J, Selvakumar S, How TV, Bakran A. Factors associated with early failure of arteriovenous fistulae for hemodialysis access. *Eur J Vasc Endovasc Surg* 1996; **12**: 207–213.
13. Patel NH, Revanur VK, Khanna A *et al.* Vascular access for hemodialysis : an in-depth review. *J Nephrol* 2001; **14**: 146–156.
14. Yerdel MA, Kesenci M, Yazicioglu KM, Doseyen Z, Turkcapar AG, Anadol E. Effect of haemodynamic variables on surgically created arteriovenous fistula flow. *Nephrol Dial Transplant* 1997; **12**: 1684–1688.
15. Rodriguez JA, Armadans L, Ferrer E *et al.* The function of permanent vascular access. *Nephrol Dial Transplant* 2000; **15**: 402–408.
16. Ikegaya N, Yamamoto T, Takeshita A *et al.* Elevated erythropoietin receptor and transforming growth factor in stenotic arteriovenous fistula used for hemodialysis. *J Am Soc Nephrol* 2000; **11**: 928–935.
17. Sands JJ, Ferrel LM, Perry MA. The role of color flow Doppler in dialysis access [Abstract]. *Semin Nephrol* 2002; **22**: 195–201.
18. El Minshawy O, El Aziz TA, El Ghani HA. Evaluation of vascular access complications in acute and chronic haemodialysis. *J Vasc Access* 2004; **5**: 76–82.

19. Kim OY, Yang CW, Yoon AS *et al*. Blood flow as a predictor of early failures of native arteriovenous fistulas in hemodialysis patients. *Am J Nephrol* 2001; **21**: 221–225.
20. Roy-Chaudhury P, Duncan H, Barrett W *et al*. Vascular brachytherapy for hemodialysis vascular access dysfunction: exploring an unmet clinical need. *Invasive Cardiol* 2003; **15 (Suppl A)**: 25A–30A.
21. Reisman M, Gray WA. Vascular brachytherapy and the strontium-90 vascular brachytherapy system. *J Invasive Cardiol* 2003; **15**: 520–523.
22. Duncan H, Ferguson L, Faris I. Incidence of the radial steal syndrome in patients with brescia fistula for haemodialysis: its clinical significance [Abstract]. *J Vasc Surg* 1986; **4**: 144–147.
23. Zibari GB, Rohr MS, Landreneau MD *et al*. Complications from permanent hemodialysis vascular access. *Surgery* 1988; **104**: 681–686.
24. Goff CD, Sato DT, Bloch PH *et al*. Steal syndrome complicating access procedures: can it be predicted? *Ann Vasc Surg* 2000; **14**: 138–144.
25. Schanzer H, Schwartz M, Harrington E *et al*. Treatment of ischemia due to steal by arteriovenous fistula with distal artery ligation and revascularization. *J Vasc Surg* 1988; **7**: 770–773.
26. Haimov M, Schanzer F, Skladani M. Pathogenesis and management of upper-extremity ischemia following angioaccess surgery. *Blood Purif* 1996; **14**: 350–354.
27. Reyal Y, Robinson C, Salama A, Levy JB. Neurological complications from brachial arteriovenous fistulae. *Nephrol Dial Transplant* 2004; **19**: 1923–1924.
28. Abbott KC, Trespalacio S, Agodoa LY. Arteriovenous fistula use and heart disease in long-term haemodialysis patients: analysis of United States renal data system morbidity and mortality wave II. *J Nephrol* 2003; **16**: 822–830.
29. Amerling R, Malostovker I, Dubrow A *et al*. High output heart failure in patients with upper arm A–V fistulae: diagnosis and treatment. *Hemodial Int* 2005; **9**: 70–71.
30. Wijen E, Keuter XH, Planken NR *et al*. The relation between vascular access flow and different types of vascular access with systemic hemodynamics in hemodialysis patients. *Artif Organs* 2005; **29**:960–964.
31. Witz M, Werner M, Bernheim J *et al*. Ultrasound-guided compression repair of pseudoaneurysms complicating a forearm dialysis arteriovenous fistula. *Nephrol Dial Transplant* 2000; **15**: 1453–1454.
32. Rabindranauth P, Shindelman L. Transluminal stent-graft repair for pseudoaneurysm of PTFE hemodialysis grafts. *J Endovasc Surg* 1998; **5**: 138–141.
33. Nassar GM, Ayus JC. Infectious complications of the haemodialysis access. *Kidney Int* 2001; **60**: 1–13.
34. Zibari GB, Gadallah MF, Landreneau M *et al*. Preoperative vancomycin prophylaxis decreases incidence of postoperative haemodialysis vascular access infections. *Am J Kidney Dis* 1997; **30**: 343–348.
35. Mohamed M, Habte-Gabr E, Mueller W. Infected arteriovenous hemodialysis graft presenting as left and right infective endocarditis. *Am J Nephrol* 1995; **15**: 521–523.
36. Nakhoul F, Yigla M, Gilman R, Reiner SA, Abassi Z. The pathogenesis of pulmonary hypertension in haemodialysis patients via arterio-venous access. *Nephrol Dial Transplant* 2005; **20**: 1686–1692.

M.P. Senthil Kumar Irving Taylor

14

Review of recent randomised clinical trials in surgery

Good quality, randomised, clinical trials seek to eliminate bias and provide objective evidence of effectiveness of interventions. Though there are a number of logistic issues pertaining to subjecting surgical procedures to randomised clinical trials and their subsequent interpretation of the results sometimes complex, they still remain one of the best ways of assessing competing therapeutic options or evaluating newer therapies against a gold standard. Randomised, clinical trials rank high in the hierarchy of evidence and are vital resources in everyday practice, in the current era of evidence based surgery. This chapter summarises the background, methodology and outcomes of a selection of randomised trials in various surgical specialities in the last couple of years. 'Key points' aim to summarise the message from the study or outline the potential impact that the study results may have on clinical practice.

HERNIA SURGERY

A number of fundamental questions pertaining to the management of hernias continue to be raised and some have been addressed by recent randomised trials.

ASYMPTOMATIC HERNIAS – TO TREAT OR OBSERVE

The annual incidence of adverse events ('hernia accidents') such as strangulation and intestinal obstruction in the natural history of inguinal hernias is estimated

M.P. Senthil Kumar MS FRCS(Ed)
Specialist Registrar in Surgery, University College London Hospital, London, UK
E-mail: sanskrity@hotmail.com

Irving Taylor MD ChM FRCS FMedSci FRCPS(Glasg) (for correspondence)
David Patey Professor of Surgery and Vice-Dean & Director of clinical studies, Royal Free and University College Medical School, 4th Floor, The Medical School Building, 74 Huntley Street, London WC1E 6AU, UK, E-mail: irving.taylor@ucl.ac.uk

to be as low as 3 per 1000 patients.[1] The operative mortality for hernias in the event of the above complications is also very low. Given that elective hernia repair carries morbidity such as infection, haematoma, severe groin pain, testicular atrophy and recurrence, there may be a role for conservative management of selected inguinal hernias.

A multicentre, North American study[2] randomised a total of 720 men with asymptomatic or minimally symptomatic inguinal hernias (no hernia-related pain limiting normal activities; no history of irreducibility in the preceding 6 weeks) into an observation arm (364 patients) and a treatment arm (356 patients; open Liechtenstein's repair). Follow-up was from 2–4.5 years with the primary outcome measures being pain interfering with activity and the change from baseline of the physical component score (PCS) of the Short Form-36 (quality-of-life tool) at 2 years.

Primary intention-to-treat outcomes were similar at 2 years for watchful waiting and surgical repair: pain interfering with activities (5.1% versus 2.2%, respectively; $P = 0.52$); improvement over baseline of PCS (0.29 points versus 0.13 points; $P = 0.79$). One watchful-waiting patient (0.3%) experienced acute hernia incarceration without strangulation within 2 years; a second had acute incarceration with bowel obstruction at 4 years, giving a frequency of 1.8/1000 patient-years.

However, the major limitation of the study is the potential selection bias which limits its generalisability (the study was limited to privately insured patients; 2350 of 3074 patients screened were excluded because they were either ineligible or refused consent and the inclusion criteria could well be interpreted subjectively). The short duration of follow-up and a high cross-over rate to the operative arm are the other limitations.

WHICH OPERATION?

The Shouldice operation is the gold standard technique for open non-mesh hernia repair with low recurrence rates. Laparoscopic hernia repair is still evolving and some reports tend to suggest a high recurrence rate in the long term.

A Swedish multicentre trial[3] has reported the 5-year results of a randomised comparison of the Shouldice repair with laparoscopic transabdominal preperitoneal patch (TAPP) repair for primary inguinal hernia. There were 454 patients in the TAPP group and 466 in the Shouldice group who completed the 5-year follow-up. All procedures were performed by trained surgeons. While the recurrence rates were similar – 6.6% for Shouldice and 6.7% for TAPP – it is to be noted that these rates are high when compared to the generally reported rates for open mesh repair.

WHICH MESH?

Chronic inguinal pain of varying grades is an important potential adverse effect of open inguinal hernia repair and occurs in about a third of all patients undergoing open inguinal hernia surgery, with about 3% of all patients suffering severe pain.

A multicentre, randomised trial[4] compared the impact on chronic pain of a conventional heavy-weight prolene mesh (pore size 1 mm; weight 85 g/m^2)

with that of a light-weight mesh composed of prolene and polyglactin (pore size 4 mm; weight after absorption 32 g/m^2). The pre-operative incidence of nerve identification and injury were comparable. Questionnaire data relating to incidence and severity of pain (visual analogue score) and activity were collected at 1, 3 and 12 months. Of the total of 330 patients randomised, 135 in the light-weight group and 125 patients in the heavy-weight group were available for analysis at 12-month follow-up. While the incidence of pain was similar in both groups at 1 and 3 months, it was significantly higher in the heavy-weight mesh group (51.6%) than the light-weight mesh group (39.5%) at 12 months ($P = 0.03$, Fisher's exact test). There was no significant difference in the mean pain scores between the groups at 1 and 3 months. The incidence of severe or very severe pain at 12 months was similar in either group (3% in light-weight versus 4% in heavy-weight groups). While the time to return to normal activities was similar, there was a higher incidence of recurrence of hernia at 12 months in the light-weight group (5.6%) than the heavy-weight group (0.7%; $P = 0.03$, Fisher's exact test].

Repair of incisional hernias with standard polypropylene mesh reduces recurrence rates when compared to suture repairs, but may be associated with serious surgical site infections, patient discomfort, restriction of abdominal wall mobility and fistulae. Light-weight and large pore composite meshes may improve the functional properties and reduce local complications.

A multicentre, European trial[5] randomised 83 patients with incisional hernia to the light-weight composite mesh arm and 82 patients to the standard polypropylene or polyester mesh arm. Complications, recurrence rates and quality of life were assessed for up to 24 months. There were no differences in physical function and daily activities scores at any point in time. Postoperative complication rates were comparable. However, the light-weight mesh group had a trend towards higher rate of recurrence at 17% when compared to the standard mesh (7%). Though the differences in recurrence rates failed to reach statistical significance ($P = 0.052$, Cochran-Mantel-Haenszel test), this must be interpreted in the light of the fact that the study was underpowered.

A number of alternatives to the standard Lichtenstein mesh patch continue to be developed. One randomised trial[6] recruiting 300 patients evaluated a three component bilayer prolene mesh device, the Prolene Hernia System (PHS), which involves minimal or no suturing for anchorage. Both short-term (operative time, pain, return to activity) and long-term outcomes (chronic pain, recurrence) were evaluated with follow-up visits at 1 week, 1 month and 1 year. The PHS repair was quicker by 10 minutes ($P < 0.001$). There were no significant differences between the groups in postoperative pain, analgesic requirements, hospital stay, complications, chronic pain and return to work or sporting activities. There were no recurrences in either group at 1 year.

Key point 1

- Delaying surgical repair of inguinal hernias in men, until symptoms are significant, appears to be a safe approach. Watchful waiting is an acceptable management option for men with minimally symptomatic inguinal hernias.

Key point 2–5

- The transabdominal preperitoneal patch (TAPP) repair is associated with a recurrence rate comparable to the Shouldice technique at 5 years of follow-up.

- Light-weight mesh used at open inguinal hernioplasty has a lower incidence of chronic inguinal pain at 1 year, but a higher recurrence rate of hernia when compared to heavy-weight mesh.

- In incisional hernia repair, postoperative complications and quality-of-life scores up to 2 years' postoperatively are comparable for light-weight composite mesh and the standard heavy-weight mesh. Use of a light-weight composite mesh may have a higher recurrence rate.

- Inguinal hernia repair using the Prolene Hernia System is quicker to perform when compared to Lichtenstein repair. The ease of convalescence, pain, complications and recurrence rates up to 1 year are comparable.

HEPATOPANCREATICOBILIARY SURGERY

HEPATOCELLULAR CARCINOMA

Traditionally, resection has been the preferred approach to hepatocellular carcinomas. Two recent. randomised trials have suggested that non-resective alternatives may be equally effective for small hepatocellular carcinomas.

One study from Taiwan[7] randomised a total of 76 patients with one or two hepatocellular carcinomas less than 3 cm in size, to surgical resection ($n = 38$) or percutaneous ethanol injection ($n = 38$). Follow-up ranged from 12–59 months. Main outcome measures were recurrence rates and overall survival. There were 15 recurrences and 5 deaths in the surgical resection group compared to 18 recurrences and 3 deaths in the percutaneous ethanol group. By Kaplan-Meier analysis, the 1–5-year survival rates were 97.4%, 91.3%, 88.1%, 88.1%, and 81.8% for the resection group and 100%, 100%, 96.7%, 92.1%, and 46% for the percutaneous ethanol group, respectively. These differences were not statistically significant.

In a Chinese study,[8] patients with a solitary hepatocellular carcinoma less than 5 cm were randomised and treated by segmental resection ($n = 90$) or percutaneous local ablative therapy ($n = 71$) which involved radiofrequency ablation. The 1-, 2-, 3-, and 4-year overall survival rates after surgery and percutaneous ablation and were 93.3%, 82.3%, 73.4%, 64.0% and 95.8%, 82.1%, 71.4%, 67.9%, respectively. The corresponding disease-free survival rates were 86.6%, 76.8%, 69%, 51.6% and 85.9%, 69.3%, 64.1%, 46.4%, respectively. Statistically, there was no difference between these two treatments.

The conclusion from these studies is that the surgical and local ablative therapies studied are equally effective and that both these options may be considered as first-line treatments in small hepatocellular carcinomas.

However, the relatively small numbers of patients and the short duration of follow-up are limitations of both the studies.

PANCREATECTOMY

Pylorus preservation in pancreaticoduodenectomy has the advantage of reduced operative time, intra-operative blood loss and easier postoperative endoscopic access to the biliary tree when compared to the standard Whipple operation. Evidence on superiority of either of these procedures on other aspects such as postoperative recovery, gastric function and oncological outcomes is unclear.

One randomised study[9] has reported on the short- and long-term outcomes of pylorus preserving pancreaticoduodenectomy (PPPD) compared to Whipple resection for pancreatic and peri-ampullary tumours. There were 53 evaluable patients in the PPPD group and 57 patients in the Whipple group. Follow-up ranged from 4–93 months (median, 63.1 months). Though the operative time and blood loss were less in the PPPD group, there were no differences in the peri-operative mortality or overall morbidity (including delayed gastric emptying). At 6 months, the capacity to work was better with PPPD (77% for PPPD versus 56% for Whipple; $P = 0.019$). Long-term outcomes including recurrence, survival, weight gain and quality of life were identical.

Delayed gastric emptying (DGE), thought to be partly due to a prolonged gastroparesis of multifactorial aetiology, in the first few weeks after pancreaticoduodenectomy is a difficult complication to manage. Some studies have suggested that DGE may be more common after PPPD than a standard Whipple operation, while others have found no difference. One recent study[10] has addressed the effect of the type of duodenojejunostomy (retrocolic versus antecolic) on the incidence of DGE after PPPD for peri-ampullary and bile duct tumours.

There were 20 patients in each of the two arms. DGE, which was the main outcome measure, was defined as: (i) prolonged aspiration of > 500 ml/day from a nasogastric tube left in place for > 10 days; (ii) need for re-insertion of a nasogastric tube; or (iii) failure of unlimited oral intake by the 14th postoperative day. DGE occurred in 5% of patients with the antecolic route for duodenojejunostomy versus 50% with the retrocolic route ($P = 0.0014$). Those with the antecolic route had a significantly shorter duration of postoperative nasogastric tube drainage (4.2 days versus 18.9 days), and shorter hospital stay (28 days versus 48 days) when compared to those with the retrocolic anastomosis. By postoperative day 14, all patients with the antecolic route could take solid foods, while only 55% of the patients with the retrocolic route could take solid foods ($P = 0.0007$).

PERI-OPERATIVE CARE

Postoperative nausea and vomiting after laparoscopic cholecystectomy can delay recovery and discharge. An Italian double-blind, placebo-controlled, randomised trial[11] has reported on the usefulness of a single pre-operative dose of dexamethasone. Forty-nine patients were randomised to receive an 8-mg dose of dexamethasone intravenously before surgery while 52 patients received a placebo. Outcome measures were postoperative nausea and vomiting, pain, analgesic and anti-emetic requirements in the first 24 hours postoperatively. Seven patients (14%) in the dexamethasone group reported nausea and vomiting compared to 24 patients (46%) in the placebo group ($P = 0.001$). The proportion of patients requiring anti-emetics was significantly higher in the placebo group (44%) compared to the dexamethasone group (10%). There were no differences in postoperative pain scores or analgesic requirements.

In the setting of laparoscopic cholecystectomy, another randomised trial.[12] in a three group parallel design, compared pre-operative fasting (which is standard practice) with intake of 800 ml of a carbohydrate rich drink (50 kcal/100 ml) the evening before surgery and 400 ml 2 hours before surgery and a placebo group. There were 58 patients in the fasted group, 59 in the placebo group and 55 patients in the carbohydrate drink group. The incidence of postoperative nausea and vomiting between 12 and 24 hours was significantly lower in the carbohydrate drink group when compared to the fasted group. Though the study suffers from a small sample size and the mechanism of the effect is not clear, it is worth exploring the effect in a larger study in the current era of multimodal optimisation.

Key point 6–9

- For small hepatocellular carcinomas, percutaneous ethanol injection and radiofrequency ablation appear to be as effective as standard surgical resection.

- When compared to standard Whipple operation, pylorus preserving pancreaticoduodenectomy (PPPD) has certain intra-operative advantages. Peri-operative morbidity and mortality, long-term oncological and quality-of-life outcomes are, however, similar.

- Delayed gastric emptying after pylorus preserving pancreaticoduodenectomy occurs less often after an antecolic duodenojejunostomy than a retrocolic anastomosis.

- In laparoscopic cholecystectomy, a single pre-operative 8-mg dose of dexamethasone appears to be effective in reducing the incidence of postoperative nausea and vomiting. Pre-operative administration of a carbohydrate-rich drink as compared to overnight fasting may also have a beneficial effect on postoperative nausea and vomiting.

UPPER GASTROINTESTINAL SURGERY

GASTRO-OESOPHAGEAL REFLUX DISEASE

Fundoplication and proton pump inhibitor (PPI) therapy are established treatment methods for gastro-oesophageal reflux disease (GORD). While open fundoplication has been compared with medical therapy in randomised trials, it is only recently that a study[13] has compared the outcomes of laparoscopic fundoplication with maximal medical therapy.

A total of 217 patients with symptomatic GORD of more than 6 months' duration were randomised to PPI therapy (n = 108) or laparoscopic Nissen fundoplication (LNF; n = 109). At 3 months, though the mean DeMeester score improved significantly in both groups when compared to their respective baseline values, only the LNF group showed a significant increase in lower oesophageal pressure. At 12 months, the mean gastrointestinal symptom rating score and the psychological general well-being index showed a greater improvement in the LNF group than the PPI group. The differences between the groups were statistically significant.

OESOPHAGOGASTRIC CANCER

With the proven beneficial effect of current chemotherapeutic agents in improving survival outcomes in advanced and inoperable gastric adenocarcinoma, there has been an increasing enthusiasm in exploring the value of initial chemotherapy (neo-adjuvant and peri-operative) even in operable oesophagogastric adenocarcinoma.

In a recent trial,[14] patients with operable adenocarcinoma involving the stomach, oesophagogastric junction or lower oesophagus were randomised to either surgery alone (n = 253) or routine peri-operative chemotherapy (combination of epirubicin, cisplatin and infusional 5-fluorouracil – 3 cycles pre-operatively followed by surgery and then 3 cycles of postoperative chemotherapy). The primary outcome measure was overall survival. Median follow-up was 4 years. Peri-operative morbidity and 30-day mortality were similar for both groups. When compared to the initial surgery group, the peri-operative chemotherapy group had a higher likelihood of overall survival (hazard ratio for death, 0.75; 95% CI, 0.60–0.93; P = 0.009). The 5-year survival rate was 36% for the peri-operative chemotherapy group versus 23% for the surgery group. Progression-free survival was also better for the peri-operative chemotherapy group (hazard ratio for progression, 0.66; 95% CI, 0.53–0.81; P < 0.001).

Key point 10 & 11

- In patients with symptomatic gastro-oesophageal reflux disease, laparoscopic Nissen fundoplication is superior to best medical management as measured by gastrointestinal symptom rating index and psychological general well-being index at 1 year.

- In operable adenocarcinoma of the stomach, oesophagogastric junction and the lower oesophagus, compared to surgery alone, peri-operative chemotherapy confers a significant survival advantage without increasing peri-operative morbidity or mortality.

COLORECTAL SURGERY

LAPAROSCOPIC COLORECTAL SURGERY

Laparoscopic surgery has been shown to confer a number of advantages including early recovery, better pain control and reduced hospital stay, when compared to conventional open surgery in many clinical contexts. Since the initial reports of laparoscopic colorectal surgery in 1992, many non-randomised trials have confirmed the safety of this approach. In the last few years, a few randomised controlled trials have provided level I evidence, comparing open and laparoscopic colorectal surgery.

The CLASSIC trial (Conventional versus Laparoscopic-Assisted Surgery In patients with Colorectal Cancer), a multicentre trial conducted over 6 years with 27 participating UK centres, has reported on short-term outcomes.[15] These include pathological outcomes (which reflect the quality and oncological soundness of surgery) as well as clinical outcomes such as morbidity and in-hospital mortality. A cohort of 253 patients received open surgery (OS) and 484 patients laparoscopically assisted surgery (LAS), of whom 29% were eventually converted to open surgery. Analysis was by intention-to-treat. There were no significant differences between the treatment arms in the proportion of Dukes' C2 tumours [7% OS; 6% LAS] and positive circumferential resection margins (CRM) for colon cancers [5% OS; 7% LAS]. Though the proportion with positive CRM for rectal cancer as a whole was similar [14% OS; 16% LAS], among those who underwent anterior resection, CRM positivity was higher in the LAS group (12%) than the OS group (6%). There were no differences in the in-hospital mortality [5% OS; 4% LAS], intra-operative complications or 30-day morbidity.

MECHANICAL BOWEL PREPARATION

Mechanical bowel preparation and antibiotic prophylaxis have traditionally been used in colorectal surgery to reduce infective postoperative complications. While there is good evidence for the effectiveness of antibiotics, the value of mechanical bowel preparation has been questioned in many prospective studies. One recent randomised trial has specifically studied the value of mechanical bowel preparation in left-sided colonic resection with primary anastomosis.[16]

Patients scheduled for elective left-sided colorectal resection with primary anastomosis were randomised to pre-operative mechanical bowel preparation (MBP) with 3 litres of polyethylene glycol (n = 78) or no mechanical bowel preparation (n = 75). All patients received antibiotic prophylaxis. The overall rate of abdominal infectious complications (anastomotic leak, intra-abdominal abscess, peritonitis and wound infection) was 22% in the MBP group and 8% in those without bowel preparation (P = 0.021). Extra-abdominal morbidity rates were significantly higher and mean hospital stay longer in those who had mechanical bowel preparation.

PILONIDAL SINUS

Simple excision of pilonidal sinus carries a high incidence of wound-related complications and a recurrence rate of up to 42%. Many alternatives such as the Bascom technique, the Karydakis flap, the Limberg flap and their modifications have been shown to achieve superior results in many case series. A Turkish study[17] has provided class I evidence in favour of the Limberg flap technique which involves a rhomboid excision of the sinus and a local rotation flap. A total of 200 consecutive patients with primary sacrococcygeal pilonidal sinus were randomised to standard simple excision and primary closure (n = 100) or Limberg flap closure (n = 100). The operative time was longer for the Limberg flap; however, the postoperative pain was significantly less, mobilisation earlier, hospital stay shorter, time to resumption of work shorter and postoperative complications fewer for the Limberg flap group compared to the primary closure group. During a median follow-up period of 28 months, there were no recurrences in the Limberg flap group compared to 11 recurrences in the simple excision and primary closure group (P = 0.001).

> ## Key point 12–14
>
> - Laparoscopically assisted surgery for colon cancer produces similar oncopathological and short-term clinical outcomes as conventional open surgery. In rectal cancer, laparoscopically assisted anterior resection needs further evaluation.
>
> - Mechanical bowel preparation does not reduce the incidence of infectious postoperative complications in left-sided colonic surgery.
>
> - Rhomboid excision and Limberg flap closure is superior to simple excision and primary closure in primary sacrococcygeal pilonidal sinus.

BREAST SURGERY AND ENDOCRINE THERAPY

SENTINEL LYMPH NODE MAPPING

Sentinel lymph node (SLN) biopsy is an acceptably accurate method of staging the axilla in breast cancer, though the optimal mapping method is being evaluated. One study from Hong Kong[18] has compared blue dye injection alone with combined radioisotope and blue dye in localising sentinel nodes. Fifty-seven women had blue dye localisation while 61 had combined mapping. All women had axillary clearance after the biopsy. The SLN was identified successfully in all 61 patients (100%) who underwent the combined technique but only in 86% of patients in the blue-dye only group. This difference was statistically significant. The accuracy and false negative rates for the identified SLN was similar in either group. The combination of blue dye and radioisotope-directed biopsy of the sentinel node seems to be the ideal technique at present.

ENDOCRINE THERAPY IN POSTMENOPAUSAL BREAST CANCER

In postmenopausal women with oestrogen receptor positive localised breast cancer, postoperative tamoxifen has been the standard adjuvant endocrine treatment. However, intolerance and recurrence rates despite 5 years of treatment leave room for improvement. Are newer agents such as the aromatase inhibitor anastrazole better? The ATAC trial[19] (Arimidex, Tamoxifen, Alone or in Combination) recruiting 9366 patients has specifically addressed this question. There were initially three arms in the trial – anastrazole only, tamoxifen only and a combination therapy arm. The combination therapy arm was closed as after an interim analysis it was felt that the combination was unlikely to show a significant benefit and that retaining this additional arm would reduce the overall power of the study. At the completion of the trial there were 3092 patients in the anastrazole and 3094 patients in the tamoxifen group. After a median follow-up of 68 months, the anastrazole group had a significantly prolonged disease-free survival (hazard ratio 0.87; 95% CI 0.78–0.97; $P = 0.01$); significantly reduced distant metastasis (hazard ratio 0.86; 95% CI 0.74–0.99; $P = 0.04$); significantly lower incidence of contralateral cancers (relative risk reduction of 42%; 95% CI 12–62%). Anastrazole also had fewer side effects, especially gynaecological and vascular, but there was a higher incidence of arthralgia and fractures.

THYROIDECTOMY AND CENTRAL NECK DISSECTION – TO DRAIN OR NOT TO DRAIN

The notion of selective drainage of the operative space after thyroidectomy is not new. Drainage is generally performed if the dead space is large (large thyroid, extensive dissection, associated cervical lymphadenectomy), presence of a substernal goitre or an unusually hypervascular gland. A recent randomised study from Korea[20] has explored the safety of drainless thyroid surgery including in its cohort a subset of patients who in addition had central cervical lymphadenectomy (level VI). The 'drain' arm of the study ($n = 101$) had 41 hemithyroidectomies, 28 total thyroidectomies and 32 total thyroidectomies with central node dissection, while the respective numbers for the 'no drains' arm ($n = 97$) were 42, 18 and 37. The mean duration to drain removal was 4.8 days. There were no significant differences in the overall locoregional postoperative complications between the drained group (6.9%) and the undrained group (10.3%). Subset analysis of those subjected to neck dissection did not reveal any significant differences either. Hospital stay was significantly less for the undrained group (mean of 9.3 days for drain group and 6.8 days for no-drain group; $P < 0.05$).

The shortfalls of the study are: (i) the inclusion of patients who underwent thyroidectomy alone alongside those who also had neck dissection; (ii) not using stratified randomisation; and (iii) the relatively small numbers who underwent neck dissection. Nevertheless, the study does highlight the feasibility of avoiding drainage in patients undergoing thyroidectomy and central neck dissection.

Key point 15–17

- Combined mapping with blue dye and radioisotope is better than blue dye alone in localising SLN in the axilla.

- Anastrazole should be preferred over tamoxifen as the endocrine treatment of choice in the adjuvant treatment of oestrogen receptor positive localised breast cancer in postmenopausal women.

- Thyroidectomy with central cervical lymphadenectomy is feasible and safe without the use of drainage. Not draining the surgical space significantly reduces hospital stay.

Key points for clinical practice

- Delaying surgical repair of inguinal hernias in men, until symptoms are significant, appears to be a safe approach. Watchful waiting is an acceptable management option for men with minimally symptomatic inguinal hernias.

- The transabdominal preperitoneal patch (TAPP) repair is associated with a recurrence rate comparable to the Shouldice technique at 5 years of follow-up.

- Light-weight mesh used at open inguinal hernioplasty has a lower incidence of chronic inguinal pain at 1 year, but a higher recurrence rate of hernia when compared to heavy-weight mesh.

- In incisional hernia repair, postoperative complications and quality-of-life scores up to 2 years' postoperatively are comparable for light-weight composite mesh and the standard heavy-weight mesh. Use of a light-weight composite mesh may have a higher recurrence rate.

- Inguinal hernia repair using the Prolene Hernia System is quicker to perform when compared to Lichtenstein repair. The ease of convalescence, pain, complications and recurrence rates up to 1 year are comparable.

- For small hepatocellular carcinomas, percutaneous ethanol injection and radiofrequency ablation appear to be as effective as standard surgical resection.

- When compared to standard Whipple operation, pylorus preserving pancreaticoduodenectomy (PPPD) has certain intra-operative advantages. Peri-operative morbidity and mortality, long-term oncological and quality-of-life outcomes are, however, similar.

- Delayed gastric emptying after pylorus preserving pancreaticoduodenectomy occurs less often after an antecolic duodenojejunostomy than a retrocolic anastomosis.

- In laparoscopic cholecystectomy, a single pre-operative 8-mg dose of dexamethasone appears to be effective in reducing the incidence of postoperative nausea and vomiting. Pre-operative administration of a carbohydrate-rich drink as compared to overnight fasting may also have a beneficial effect on postoperative nausea and vomiting.

- In patients with symptomatic gastro-oesophageal reflux disease, laparoscopic Nissen fundoplication is superior to best medical management as measured by gastrointestinal symptom rating index and psychological general well-being index at 1 year.

- In operable adenocarcinoma of the stomach, oesophagogastric junction and the lower oesophagus, compared to surgery alone, peri-operative chemotherapy confers a significant survival advantage without increasing peri-operative morbidity or mortality.

(continued)

Key points for clinical practice

- Laparoscopically assisted surgery for colon cancer produces similar oncopathological and short-term clinical outcomes as conventional open surgery. In rectal cancer, laparoscopically assisted anterior resection needs further evaluation.

- Mechanical bowel preparation does not reduce the incidence of infectious postoperative complications in left-sided colonic surgery.

- Rhomboid excision and Limberg flap closure is superior to simple excision and primary closure in primary sacrococcygeal pilonidal sinus.

- Combined mapping with blue dye and radioisotope is better than blue dye alone in localising SLN in the axilla.

- Anastrazole should be preferred over tamoxifen as the endocrine treatment of choice in the adjuvant treatment of oestrogen receptor positive localised breast cancer in postmenopausal women.

- Thyroidectomy with central cervical lymphadenectomy is feasible and safe without the use of drainage. Not draining the surgical space significantly reduces hospital stay.

References

1. Neutra R, Velez A, Ferrada R, Galan R. Risk of incarceration of inguinal hernia in Cali, Colombia. *J Chronic Dis* 1981; **34**: 561–564.
2. Fitzgibbons Jr RJ, Giobbie-Harder A, Gibbs JO *et al*. Watchful waiting versus repair of inguinal hernia in minimally symptomatic men: a randomized clinical trial. *JAMA* 2006; **285**: 285–297.
3. Arvidsson D, Berndsen FH, Larsson LG *et al*. Randomised clinical trial comparing 5-year recurrence rate after laparoscopic versus Shouldice repair of primary inguinal hernia. *Br J Surg* 2005; **92**: 1085–1091.
4. O'Dwyer PJ, Kingsnorth AN, Molloy RG *et al*. Randomised clinical trial assessing impact of a light weight or heavyweight mesh on chronic pain after inguinal hernia. *Br J Surg* 2005; **92**: 166–170.
5. Conze J, Kingsnorth AN, Flament JB *et al*. Randomised clinical trial comparing lightweight composite mesh with polyester or polypropylene mesh for incisional hernia repair. *Br J Surg* 2005; **92**: 1488–1493.
6. Vironen J, Nieminen J, Eklund A, Paavolainen P. Randomised clinical trial of Lichtenstein patch or prolene hernia system for inguinal hernia repair. *Br J Surg* 2006; **93**: 33–39.
7. Huang G, Lee P, Tsang Y *et al*. Percutaneous ethanol injection versus surgical resection for the treatment of small hepatocellular carcinoma: a prospective study. *Ann Surg* 2005; **242**: 36–42.
8. Chen M, Li J, Zheng Y *et al*. A prospective randomized trial comparing percutaneous local ablative therapy and partial hepatectomy for small hepatocellular carcinoma. *Ann Surg* 2006; **243**: 321–328.
9. Seiler CA, Wagner M, Bachmann T *et al*. Randomised clinical trial of pylorus-preserving duodenopancreatectomy versus classical Whipple resection – long term results. *Br J Surg* 205; **92**: 547–556.
10. Tani M, Terasawa H, Kawai M *et al*. Improvement of delayed gastric emptying in pylorus-preserving pancreaticoduodenectomy: results of a prospective, randomized,

controlled trial. *Ann Surg* 2006; **243**: 316–320.

11. Feo CV, Sortini D, Ragazzi R. Randomised clinical trial of the effect of pre-operative dexamethasone on nausea and vomiting after laparoscopic cholecystectomy. *Br J Surg* 2006; **93**: 295–299.

12. Hausel J, Nygren J, Thorell M *et al*. Randomised clinical trial of the effects of oral preoperative carbohydrates on postoperative nausea and vomiting after laparoscopic cholecystectomy. *Br J Surg* 2005; **92**: 415–421.

13. Mahon D, Rhodes M, Decadt B *et al*. Randomised clinical trial of laparoscopic Nissen fundoplication compared with proton-pump inhibitors for treatment of chronic gastro-oesophageal reflux. *Br J Surg* 2005; **92**: 695–699.

14. Cunningham D, Allum WH, Stenning SP *et al*. Perioperative chemotherapy versus surgery alone for resectable gastroesophageal cancer. *N Engl J Med* 2006; **355**: 11–20.

15. Guillou PJ, Quirke P, Thorpe H, Walker J, Smith AMH, Brown JM. Short-term end points of conventional versus laparoscopic –assisted surgery in patients with colorectal cancer (MRC CLASSIC trial): multicentre, randomised controlled trial. *Lancet* 2005; **365**: 1718–1726.

16. Bucher P, Gervaz P, Soravia C. Randomised clinical trial of mechanical bowel preparation versus no preparation before elective left-sided colorectal surgery. *Br J Surg* 2005; **92**: 409–414.

17. Akca T, Colak T, Ustunsoy B. Randomised clinical trial comparing primary closure with the Limberg flap in the treatment of primary sacrococcygeal pilonidal disease. *Br J Surg* 2005; **92**: 1081–1084.

18. Hung WK, Chan CM, Ying M *et al*. Randomised clinical trial comparing blue dye with combined dye and isotope for sentinel lymph node biopsy in breast cancer. *Br J Surg* 2005; **92**: 1494–1497.

19. The ATAC trialists' group. Results of the ATAC (Arimidex, tamoxifen, alone or in combination) trial after completion of 5 years' adjuvant treatment for breast cancer. *Lancet* 2005; **365**: 60–62.

20. Lee SW, Choi, EC, Lee YM *et al*. Is lack of placement of drains after thyroidectomy with central neck dissection safe? A prospective, randomized study. *Laryngoscope* 2006; **116**: 1632–1635.

Index